A Rational Case for Life

Why the Unborn Matter

Randal L. N. Mandock, Ph.D.

En Route Books and Media, LLC
Saint Louis, MO

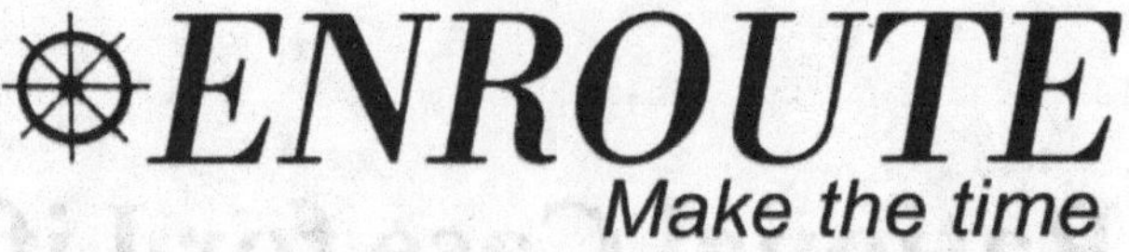

En Route Books and Media, LLC
5705 Rhodes Avenue
St. Louis, MO 63109

Contact us at contactus@enroutebooksandmedia.com

Cover art by Sebastian Mahfood using DALL-E

ISBN: 979-8-88870-410-3
Library of Congress Control Number: 2025944193

Dedication

This book is dedicated to Fr. James Buckley, FSSP, who explained to me that precision in medical terminology is just as important as precision in science, engineering, and religion.

Foreword

As a free agent (i.e., not officially representing any Church, ecclesial body, or religion), I choose to propose a method of revising definitions and terminology in the area of human pregnancy. I believe the changes inspired by this method will better serve the cause of unborn living children than the continued adoption of and acquiescence to popular notions about certain definitions and terminology used in popular accounts.

My only authority in proposing these changes rests on reason and a desire to assist medical personnel, lawyers, judges, legislators, and the devoutly religious to better position themselves to defend mothers and their unborn children. There is, however, an authority that I answer to in matters of faith and morality: the Catholic Church. The doctrinal office of this Church has charted for two millennia an inspired path between authority and reason in pursuit of its care for human souls on earth. This is evident once again in its recognition of the virtue of prudence and the value of reason in its assessment of the conditions that exist at the start of an individual person's life.

I am not a professional philosopher, theologian, bioethicist, medical specialist, or member of the clergy. I am a simple retired physical science professor who also taught religious education classes for a few decades.

Acknowledgments

Several learned individuals were involved in my decision to put into book form a topic I had been writing about and discussing for more than four decades. I would like to gratefully acknowledge their contributions here. This book would not have been possible without my discussions about three decades ago with Fr. James Buckley (of happy memory), FSSP, who first put me on the right path of understanding the power of definitions, consistency, and precision when consideration is made of pregnancy, complications of pregnancy, and induced abortion.

After a former pastor of mine did a critical review of an early draft of the book, the second person to exhaustively review the manuscript was my brother, Richard Mandock. His input, as representative of someone not well-versed in theology, resulted in simplification and more detailed explanations of some of the sections in the manuscript.

Fr. Benedict Abugu, OFM, Conv., a philosopher and bioethicist, reviewed an early copy of the manuscript and made critical suggestions for improvement. His expertise in Catholic and secular philosophy, bioethics, logic, and Catholic theology assisted me to refine several sections of the manuscript.

Fr. Brian Lorei is pastor of my parish home, St. Stephen the Martyr parish in Lilburn, Georgia. He received an early copy of the manuscript and was very supportive of the effort to increase the appeal of the pro-life message to a wider audience.

Dr. Elizabeth Rex in personal communications sharpened my understanding of the definition of pregnancy. My conversations with her caused me to revise several chapters of the book.

I thank the Institute for Theological Encounter with Science and Technology for hosting a webinar on the subject of this book, Dr. Sebastian Mahfood, OP, for arranging the webinar, Sheila Roth for webinar logistics, Francis Etheredge for co-presenting in the webinar, Dr. Kathleen Raviele for assistance with gynecological and obstetric questions, and Dr. Elizabeth Rex for constructive conversations that improved the content of my webinar presentation. The webinar is available online at http://www.faithscience.org.

A person who ultimately made publication of this book possible is Dr. Sebastian Mahfood, OP, president of En Route Books and Media. His interest and assistance converted my raw manuscript into a book to be published.

Table of Contents

Dedication....................i

Foreword....................iii

Acknowledgments....................v

Chapter 1: On Misdirection and Disinformation....................1

Chapter 2: Introduction....................5

General....................5
My Understanding of Catholic Doctrinal Authority....................18
Why I Wrote This Book....................21

Chapter 3: The Scope of the Protection of the Unborn and the Message....................23

Religious Significance of the Message....................23
Political Significance of the Message....................24
The Legitimacy of Abortion?....................25
What Makes a Religion True?....................27
Some Practical Considerations....................29

Chapter 4: On Life....................35

What is life?....................35

One Secularist Perspective 35
One Religious Perspective 36
Is Life Important? 37
One Secularist Perspective 37
One Religious Perspective 38
If Life is Important, What About Death? 39
One Secularist Perspective 39
Pascal's Wager 39
One Religious Perspective 40
One Secularist Perspective 42
One Religious Perspective 42

Chapter 5: A Brief Note on the Nature of Science and the Distinction between Physical and Biological Science 45

Introduction 45
The Contrast Between Religion and Science 45
Brief Note About the Sciences and Engineering 46
On the Physical and Biological Sciences 47
St. Augustine's Warning 54

Chapter 6: On the Conjugal Embrace and the Origin and Nature of Man 57

Male and Female He Created Them 57
One Secularist Perspective 57
Some Religious Perspectives 58

Chapter 7: On In Vitro Fertilization, Contraception, and Natural Family Planning....69

What's Wrong With In Vitro Fertilization and Contraception. 69
How to Refer to the Destruction of Nascent Human Life.......... 75
Categories of Abortion.... 79
Loss of an Unborn Child Not to be Considered an Abortion ... 80
An Ambiguity in Dignitas Personae?.... 81
Embryo Adoption.... 82
Effectiveness of In Vitro Fertilization Versus Natural Family Planning.... 83

Chapter 8: A Brief Note on the Nature of the One True God and His Relationship to Man.... 87

Chapter 9: On Doubt and Uncertainty in the Matters of Human Conception and Pregnancy.... 101

Doubt and Uncertainty in General, with Examples.... 101
A Diseased Uterus.... 105
Ectopic Pregnancy.... 109
Implantation in a Fallopian Tube.... 113
Miscarriage.... 117
Doubts About the Origin of Human Life.... 118

Chapter 10: Words Mean Things.... 129

The Dignity of One Human Life.... 129

The Three "Exceptions"........130
Elephant in the Room – A Fourth "Exception"?........133
Justification for Recognizing the Value of Preborn Human Life 137
An Attempt at New Definitions........138
A Secular Justification for a More Accurate Redefinition of Medical Terms Related to Abortion........140
Conclusion........142

Appendix: Excerpt from the Athanasian Creed that Bears on the Nature of the Trinity and the Incarnation........143
References as Cited in the Chapters 145
Chapter 3........146
Chapter 5........148

Glossary........163

References Cited in the Glossary 183

About the Author........191

CHAPTER 1

ON MISDIRECTION AND DISINFORMATION

A girl in high school found herself pregnant and didn't know what to do about it. She and her boyfriend talked to friends, a Christian group, and others. After some time, someone suggested an abortion clinic in a city far away. They went to the clinic but became convinced against having an abortion. Besides being illegal, it was not a good idea. When the girl finally went to her parents to tell them about the pregnancy, they forbade her from ever seeing her boyfriend again. A short time later, the parents changed their mind and insisted that she marry her boyfriend, who was about to leave town for military service. The two were married, but it turned out to be a bad decision for all parties.

A girl in college found herself pregnant. She did not think that having a baby at that point in her life was a good idea. How to resolve this serious problem? The news media and public educational system had her convinced that a fetus is nothing more than a piece of invasive tissue that would best be removed at her convenience. Her boyfriend tried to discourage her from having an abortion, insisting that they get married, but she was not interested in being tied down in a marriage while still in college. Besides, everyone knew that a fetus is not a legal person or even a human person—it is merely a piece of invasive tissue, like a wart, that can easily be scraped off in a doctor's office. Even though her boyfriend protested, he agreed to pay for the abortion that she insisted on having. Her boyfriend waited in the lobby while the procedure took place. How long could it take, given that the doctor was merely scraping off a piece of invasive tissue? Yet, it took a longer time than he expected it would. When the boyfriend was allowed into the room where the girlfriend was sitting, he found a scene that he could hardly have imagined when he and his girlfriend entered the doctor's office. The room was outfitted with surgical equipment and seemed like more than an outpatient examining room.

What the boyfriend first saw on entering the room was the girl sitting on a bed, groggy from general anesthesia. She was nauseous, weak, and disoriented. There was blood on the sheets, much more blood than the boyfriend had expected to see for such a simple scab removal. Actually, the boyfriend had not expected to see any blood at all. But there the blood was, staring back at him, informing him that what was removed from his girlfriend's uterus was ***not*** a scab, a piece of invasive tissue, or an infection; it was a tiny child, a nascent living human being. No one had prepared either the girl or the boyfriend for this event. All the information generally available assured them that an abortion is a simple procedure that has nothing to do with the removal of a living being, a human person fully dependent on his mother for at least the first nine months of his life inside his mother's womb. The shock of that scene just about floored the boyfriend. However, it did not take long for his anger to well up, the deception of the abortion industry being fully realized, the realization that he was actually responsible for ending a human life, and that his relationship with his church had drastically changed. Without a remedy for the guilt and the offense against

God, the eternal ramifications would be life-shattering. Fortunately, there was a remedy, and it was to be found in his church. The decision to abort the child was a bad one for all parties.

In the ensuing years, the boyfriend began to make reparations for the death of the child, the emotional affliction his former girlfriend suffered, and his supreme insult to God. He studied the crime of abortion and its moral and societal implications. He spoke out against abortion in many forums so that no one within the range of his voice would ever again be deceived about the crime against God, man, and nature. He dedicated himself to informing others of the misdirection provided by all who promote or even acquiesce to the crime of abortion. From the ancient Greeks onward, abortion has been considered one of the most grievous evils anyone could commit. The Fathers of the Catholic Church, for instance, considered it an abhorrent crime that every religion should work against.

CHAPTER 2

INTRODUCTION

General

Robert Nugent, on his "Decrevi: Determined to be Catholic" YouTube show, commented on 17 October 2025 about the recent papal exhortation, *Dilexi Te* (Pope Leo XIV, 2025). What he said is profound and directly impacts the matter of this treatise: unborn children are the poorest of the poor. They own nothing but are presumably happy in their economic poverty. They are protected, safe from the external world, and comfortable without greed or envy. If people of religion are to protect the lives and well-being of the poor, then we must begin with the most poor among us—those living children yet to be born.

What follows is a treatise on life. Life, you ask? Isn't that a very broad topic? Yes, it is, but I will try to distill the subject into points relevant to the value of human life, especially life conceived but yet to be born. The scope of this work includes science, religion, philosophy, and political considerations. The purpose is to advocate for the lives of children, both born and unborn.

This is not a scholarly treatise intended for specialists, but a mostly-informal primer written for educated persons with a serious interest in human life and an interest in, or at least a curiosity about, religion. The fundamental premise of this treatise is religious, for true religion alone has the answers to the most ultimate of questions, questions of which answers can only be approximated by philosophy, questions which are unanswerable by science, and questions which are irrelevant to the practical aims of politics. Questions answerable by true religion can include, but are certainly not limited to the following: (1) Does the God of Christianity exist? (2) Is the human soul created by this God? (3) Is material existence the limit of my responsibility to this God? (4) Can human life have any ultimate meaning apart from this God? (5) Will anybody besides this God care in 5,000 years whether I lived or died?

This treatise is built upon my Catholic understanding of intellect and will—the ability to reason, understand, and choose between good and evil, between right and wrong. Beyond the rational arguments of philosophy (reasoning about life and the universe) and empirical knowledge from nature (knowledge gained from experience instead of from reason), Catholicism depends on truth revealed by a Creator God. The truth revealed by *the* Creator God is communicated through the *deposit of faith*. This deposit consists of the Catholic *Bible* and the rituals, prayers, *sacraments* (sacred signs that can increase holiness), and way of life communicated by the Son of God to His disciples through word, deed, and example. The non-biblical elements of the deposit of faith are called the *Apostolic Tradition*—truths essentially fixed in their nature, but open to a deeper understanding as human experience broadens over time. The authoritative interpretation and applications of the Bible are the responsibility of the *Magisterium* (teaching office) of the Catholic Church ("the Church"). In the second half of the 4th century AD, the Church codified the books of the *Old Testament* (sacred Scriptures written primarily in Hebrew prior to the earthly Incarnation of the Son of God) and the books of the *New Testa-*

ment (sacred Scriptures written primarily in Greek after the Pentecostal illumination and spiritual strengthening of the Apostles chosen by God). According to Catholic belief, the Incarnation of the Son of God began at the conception of Jesus Christ in His mother's womb, as described later in this treatise (Chapter 8). The Pentecostal illumination was the enlightening of the minds of the Apostles and other disciples of Christ by God when they were hiding in fear after the crucifixion of Christ. What we refer to as the Bible is in essence the combined libraries of Old Testament books and New Testament books.

Given that much of the Bible is an indispensable source of guidance about how to understand God and how to live the best life possible, this treatise quotes liberally from it. To get a point across in the most illuminating way possible, I am accustomed to using multiple translations of the Bible in my Scriptural quotations, including interlinear translations from the original languages (primarily Hebrew and Greek). I denote these translations within the body of this work by the initials of the titles of the translations or by the full titles of the translations. Examples are: Douay Old Testament (Challoner revision), Rheims New Testament (Challoner revision), RSV (Revised Standard Version), NAB (New American Bible), etc. I often take the text of each translation from www.biblehub.com, a convenient online reference tool that makes research fast and mostly painless. I find that translations on this website agree with published Bibles in hard copy. Many translations in English are currently available on this website, as well as interlinear translations, original languages, concordances, word studies, parallel translations, and a host of other aids to understanding the meaning of biblical texts. I also cite in the references for each chapter of this work translations not included on the Biblehub website.

Before I offer my personal understanding of the Bible, its authority, and its purpose, I will offer an excerpt from the Catholic Magisterium on how to receive this sacred text. From *Dei Verbum*, Paragraphs 15-17 (Pope Paul VI, 1965):

> 15. The principal purpose to which the plan of the old covenant was directed was to prepare for the coming of Christ, the redeemer of all and of the messianic kingdom, to announce this coming by prophecy...and to indicate its meaning through various types [prefigurements]...Now the books of the Old Testament, in accordance with the state of mankind before the time of salvation established by Christ, reveal to all men the knowledge of God and of man and the ways in which God, just and merciful, deals with men. These books, though they also contain some things which are incomplete and temporary, nevertheless show us true divine pedagogy. These same books, then, give expression to a lively sense of God, contain a store of sublime teachings about God, sound wisdom about human life, and a wonderful treasury of prayers, and in them the mystery of our salvation is present in a hidden way...
>
> 16. God, the inspirer and author of both Testaments, wisely arranged that the New Testament be hidden in the Old and the Old be made manifest in the New. For, though Christ

established the new covenant in His blood…, still the books of the Old Testament with all their parts, caught up into the proclamation of the Gospel, acquire and show forth their full meaning in the New Testament…and in turn shed light on it and explain it.

17. The word of God, which is the power of God for the salvation of all who believe…, is set forth and shows its power in a most excellent way in the writings of the New Testament. For when the fullness of time arrived…, the Word was made flesh and dwelt among us in His fullness of graces and truth…Christ established the kingdom of God on earth, manifested His Father and Himself by deeds and words, and completed His work by His death, resurrection and glorious Ascension and by the sending of the Holy Spirit. Having been lifted up from the earth, He draws all men to Himself…, He who alone has the words of eternal life...This mystery had not been manifested to other generations as it was now revealed to His holy Apostles and prophets in the Holy Spirit…so that they might preach the Gospel, stir up faith in Jesus, Christ and Lord, and gather together the Church. Now the writings of the New Testament stand as a perpetual and divine witness to these realities.

My personal understanding of the Bible considers it the collection of books mentioned above which were selected by the Catholic Church as being *inspired* by God. With God as the Bible's transcendental author and inspired men as its temporal authors, the authority of the Bible is the authority given it by the Church, described above in *Dei Verbum* 17 as the *word of God* and the *power of God.* A scholarly colleague (Fr. Benedict Abugu, personal communication, 24 January 2025) reminded me that you can know an author by the words he writes, and the Bible has much to say about its principal, transcendental Author. The dual purpose of the Bible is to assist the Church to teach the world about faith in God and to teach all men a way of life that aligns with man's created nature: to be *very good.* In fact, God created all that exists in order to show forth His goodness (Catechism of the Catholic Church, nn. 293-294; Fr. D. Bouchard, personal communication, 15 August 2025). Genesis 1:31 confirms this understanding:

> God saw all the things that he had made, and they were very good.

After many years of studying, debating, and teaching the deposit of faith, my academic views about the Bible align with the excerpt above from *Dei Verbum.* However, as a practical matter, I find myself in a position of making note of a few points of distinction between the Old and New Testaments. As can be seen in the excerpt from *Dei Verbum* above, and as reiterated by Fr. Benedict (personal communication, 24 January 2025), the Old Testament can be distilled into these few words: a preparation for the Incarnation of the Son of God. This preparation consisted of what to believe (faith) and how to behave (morality). What to believe includes instructions on virtue, wisdom, and the coming of the Messiah. The accounts, stories, poetry, and prophecies found in the Old Testament often communicate a sense of what a person ought to do and what a person ought to avoid. I find that examples in the accounts, stories, and prophecies of the Old Testament of what a person ought not do may be summarized according to these four categories: (1) frequent refusals to take God at His word, (2) misplaced desires to elevate the worldly above the spiritual, (3) tension between those claiming possession of the true God and those seeking Him, and (4) warnings against paganism. Examples of what a person ought to do are just as abundant as examples of what not to do: (1) worship of God by the first people (e.g., Adam and Eve, Cain and Abel), (2) the importance before God of sacrifice, (3) faith in God by the early patriarchs (e.g., Enoch and Noah) and many of the leaders and prophets that followed (e.g., Abraham, Moses, and Elijah), (4) codification of a limited list (Steinsaltz, 2017) of positive moral directives (~178 of 613, by my count), and (5) prayers and acts of repentance, petition, thanksgiving, and praise to God. Instead of the emphasis in a significant portion of the historical books of the Old Testament on temporal dominion and tribal conquest, the New Testament is a guidebook on service and spiritual conquest of self. In the Old Testament, the presence of God was manifest in many ways, such as in the Garden of Eden, in the form of men or angels to Abraham and Jacob, as a voice to Moses from a burning bush, as thunder and lightning, on a mountain to Moses and in the Tabernacle, but also to Elijah on a mountain in a still, small voice. In the Old Testament, God's presence was often unexpected and supernatural, but in the New Testament the presence of God was in a human temple—a temple in which

God walked among men for 33 years—Jesus Christ, the Incarnation of the Second Person of the Trinity (see Chapter 8).

Some claim the Bible may be used as a science textbook. This claim is not applicable in the area of the physical and life sciences. Why? Because the intent of the authors of the various books of the Bible was religious. This can be seen in the message of the authors, the literary styles used by the authors, and the timeframe in which the biblical books were written. When contrasted against actual scientific works prior to the birth of Christ (e.g., Eratosthenes' measurement of the circumference of the earth), the gap between these secular works and the biblical text is striking. Certain particulars in the sacred history recorded in the Bible do align in certain ways with modern science, but this is primarily true because all men who venture outdoors, gaze at the sky and stars, have ever been on the water, and have ever experienced natural hazards are capable of valid observations and conclusions about the natural world.

My decision on style of articulation in this treatise is based on the following standards: (1) consistency with common usage prior to 1960, (2) consistency with other terms in the treatise, (3) accuracy and precision in meaning, (4) alignment with religious terminology when appropriate, and (5) simplicity. Terms such as "men", "man", "woman", etc., are usually cast in this work as being generic pre-1960, but specific usage is determined by the context in which these terms are used.

Wikipedia and Wiktionary are selectively cited as sources of definitions and information. I have found that scientific entries in Wikipedia mostly align with the legitimate sources cited, whereas non-scientific entries can be biased to greater or lesser extents. I would never consult Wikipedia without frequent reference to the sources cited. Wiktionary definitions can change when the popular consensus opinion or usage changes. Therefore, some of its definitions will be different today than they were a year or more ago. However, most of the time the definitions found there can serve as useful guides to the meaning of words. In the rare instance that select definitions have changed from when writing of this treatise first began (early 2023) until it ended, the date of first access is included in parentheses.

Who I am bears on the perspective behind the text of this treatise. I am not a philosopher, theologian, medical specialist, or member of the clergy. I do not speak for any church or any religion. The opinions and deductions I offer in this work are mine and mine alone. My background and experience include science, engineering, and religion.

In Chapters 4 and 6, the reader will find two perspectives: (1) secularist, and (2) religious. I do not explore every secularist perspective that exists, nor do I go into any real depth in my examples of a secularist outlook. I write from this perspective as one who was formally educated and in receipt of a salary for most his life in a secular environment. On the other hand, my outlook on reality, like that of many, is not unimodal, but bimodal. By this I mean that I operate at a recognized level of competence in both secular and religious worldviews. Since I have spent as many years in religion as in secular environments, I have found that both perspectives can enhance each other, if clarity and truth are the goals. I endeavor to align my religious perspective with nearly two millennia of Catholic teaching as understood by *orthodox* Catholicism. I emphasize *orthodox* Catholicism because during the last decade or so there seems to have arisen what I consider an unhealthy tension between objective and subjective approaches to Catholic moral understanding, assent to dogmas, and Catholic discipline.

I do not think that anything I write here is original in the sense of not having been known beforehand, but I write to clarify, inform, and lay out rational explanations in *summary* form in order to build a case for a re-specification and tightening of the terminology used to describe pregnancy and certain medical procedures that can impact unborn life in the womb. The examples used throughout the treatise were selected to help the reader relate to concepts which may seem theoretical or confusing. *The pro-life position states that all human life, including that of unborn children, is of value before God and man and therefore must be protected from harm.* The position concerning unborn children is predicated on the belief, a belief well-supported by biology and medicine, that although an unborn child is dependent on his or her mother for sustenance, protection, and comfort, this child is not an extension or part of the mother's body. The unborn child is a separate organism with its own unique genetic makeup.

When discussing matters of human life, morality is an essential consideration. In this treatise, morality is defined as ethics grounded in divine revelation. Within Catholicism, such revelation is not merely propositional but personal, being definitively disclosed in Jesus Christ—true God and true man—recognized as the only Son of God and the divine Logos. Knowledge of Christ comes from two streams originating in the same wellspring: Sacred Scripture and the Apostolic Tradition, as introduced above. I use the following working definition of the Apostolic Tradition: this Tradition consists of all that Jesus Christ said and did of eternal relevance that was handed on in non-written form by His Apostles to their successors (cf. John 20:30-31, 21:25; Acts 1:20, 20:28; 2 Timothy 1:6), and from their successors down to us under the guidance of the Catholic Church's Magisterium. My working definition of the Catholic Magisterium is this: the teaching authority of the Catholic Church that resides in the bishops in union with the pope. In as much as work of the Apostles continued after Christ's death, resurrection, and ascension into heaven, a divine Advocate (the Holy Spirit, see Chapter 8) was sent by God (John 14:26) to prompt the Apostles to remember and better understand all that Christ taught them (Pope Paul VI, 1965).

My personal criterion for moral judgment of certain medical interventions finds its origin in Hippocrates' (circa 460-370 B.C.) dictum: "do no harm". While Catholic bioethics is not derived from Hippocrates, the Hippocratic Oath found in the oldest extant version (A.D. 900-1000) does reside in the Vatican Library. Wikipedia reproduces a version dated 1595. A nearly identical parallel translation from the Greek is found in the National Library of Medicine. In this version (Greek Medicine, 2002) is seen the following promises:

> I will use those dietary regimens which will benefit my patients according to my greatest ability and judgement, and I will do no harm or injustice to them. I will not give a lethal drug to anyone if I am asked, nor will I advise such a plan;

and similarly I will not give a woman a pessary to cause an abortion. In purity and according to divine law will I carry out my life and my art.

In this oath are found the promises to do no harm, to refrain from euthanasia and abortion, to remain ethically pure, and to live and practice medicine according to *divine law*. Divine law is "that which is enacted by God and made known to man through revelation" (Slater, 1910). It is of note that these moral convictions seem universal among men of good will and date back to ancient times. Catholic teaching on these promises dates from the Apostolic age (1st century A.D.) through today.

In theological interpretations of the moral validity of certain medical interventions, I draw upon the principle of *double effect*. This principle states that it is morally permissible to perform a moral act that has two or more outcomes, one or more good and the other(s) bad. (Greater detail can be found in online sources.) Here is a summary of the conditions (Hardon, 1980) under which this principle applies:

1. The act to be done must be good in itself or at least morally indifferent.
2. The good effect must not be obtained by means of the evil effect, the evil effect being an unintended by-product.
3. The good effect must be the intention, with the evil effect being only permitted.

4. There must be a proportionately grave reason for permitting the evil effect.

I choose to write from the Catholic religious perspective because of the unbroken historical record of succession of religious leadership from the commissioning by God of the first Apostles of Jesus Christ to the Catholic episcopate of today. To the best of my knowledge, this leadership is charged with preserving and handing on the religious faith taught the first generation by Christ Himself. Over time, through persecution, disputation, clarification, disciplining, and discovery of deeper meaning, this deposit of faith has been committed to letter, liturgy, law, and pious practices of devotion such as prayer. This faith can appeal to the serious intellect because, although peppered with mysteries, it does not contradict reason in a mind attuned to God. When I reference "true religion" in the pages that follow, it would probably be better to call it "fulfilled religion", "completed religion", or "perfected religion", since several religions recognize the truth of the one God. However, in the context of this treatise, the "fulfilled" or "completed" religion is restricted to those religions which live the *four marks of the Church* (one, holy, catholic, and Apostolic).

Elements of true religion can be found in ecclesial bodies and other religions. *Orthodox Christianity*, in particular, is a sister Church "not having full communion with the Catholic Church" (CIC Canon 844), but nonetheless a Church which manifests in its holy, universal, and Apostolic character a close affinity toward the Catholic Church. See the Glossary for examples of elements of true religion.

But what about those who have never been formally exposed to the public revelation about God? Since God desires all men to find their end in His presence, those who live in societies so isolated from the modern world that the knowledge of Christ has not yet reached them are able, when moved by divine grace in faith, to worship God in truth when they act on the promptings of the Holy Spirit (see Chapter 8) in their daily lives (Pope Paul VI, 1968). This acknowledgment pertains as well to those who through no fault of their own have never grasped the message of the Gospel of Christ or who have never arrived at an explicit knowledge of God (cf. Pope Paul VI, 1964), and yet fulfill the conditions listed in the sentence above. Since the numbers of people in these situations are known only to God, the Catholic Church acts with prudence when she works to evangelize the whole world.

My Understanding of Catholic Doctrinal Authority

In 1990, I was fortunate to have stumbled upon a resource that has served me well ever since: *Fundamentals of Catholic Dogma*, by Fr. Ludwig Ott (1960). This book is a compendium of the chief doctrines of the Catholic Church and has served a multitude of priests and seminarians since its first publication. One of the most useful features of the book is its introduction, where Fr. Ott explains the concept and object of theology, the development of dogma, the theological grades of certainty, and other basics of Catholic dogmatic theology. I quote here what I consider to be the foundational principles behind assessments of the grades of theological certainty in the hierarchy of Catholic truths.

> By dogma in the strict sense is understood a truth immediately (formally) revealed by God which has been proposed by the Teaching Authority of the Church to be believed as such. ...Dogma in its strict signification is the object of both Divine Faith (Fides Divina) and Catholic faith (Fides Catholica): it is the object of Divine Faith...by reason of its Divine Revelation; it is the object of Catholic Faith...on account of its infallible doctrinal definition by the Church...
>
> ...The highest degree of certainty appertains to the immediately revealed truths...
>
> ...*Catholic truths* or *Church doctrines*, on which the infallible Teaching Authority of the Church has finally decided, are to be accepted with a faith which is based on the sole authority of the Church (fides ecclesiastica). These truths are as infallibly certain as dogmas proper.

There are also lesser grades of theological certainty which are described by Ott but will not be quoted here. Not all doctrines are infallible. Ott says this about those doctrines of lesser grades of certainty:

> With regard to the doctrinal teaching of the Church, it must be well noted that not all the assertions of the Teaching Authority of the Church on questions of faith and morals are infallible and consequently irrevocable. Only those are infallible which emanate from General Councils repre-

> senting the whole episcopate, and the Papal Decisions Ex Cathedra...The ordinary and usual form of the Papal teaching activity is not infallible. Further, the decisions of the Roman Congregations...are not infallible. Nevertheless normally they are to be accepted with an inner assent which is based on the high supernatural authority of the Holy See.

Donum Veritatis (Sacred Congregation for the Doctrine of the Faith, 1990) defines the teaching authority of the Church, or the Magisterium, as:

> the sole authentic interpreter of the Word of God, written or handed down, by virtue of the authority which it exercises in the name of Christ.

Donum Veritatis finds alignment with Fr. Ott's descriptions, as can be seen here:

> Jesus Christ promised the assistance of the Holy Spirit to the Church's Pastors so that they could fulfill their assigned task of teaching the Gospel and authentically interpreting Revelation. In particular, He bestowed on them the charism of infallibility in matters of faith and morals. This charism is manifested when the Pastors propose a doctrine as contained in Revelation and can be exercised in various ways. Thus it is exercised particularly when the bishops in union with their visible head proclaim a doctrine by a collegial act, as is the case in an ecumenical council, or when the Roman

> Pontiff, fulfilling his mission as supreme Pastor and Teacher of all Christians, proclaims a doctrine "ex cathedra".
>
> What concerns morality can also be the object of the authentic Magisterium because the Gospel, being the Word of Life, inspires and guides the whole sphere of human behavior.
>
> Divine assistance is also given to the successors of the apostles teaching in communion with the successor of Peter, and in a particular way, to the Roman Pontiff as Pastor of the whole Church, when exercising their ordinary Magisterium, even should this not issue in an infallible definition or in a "definitive" pronouncement but in the proposal of some teaching which leads to a better understanding of Revelation in matters of faith and morals and to moral directives derived from such teaching. One must therefore take into account the proper character of every exercise of the Magisterium, considering the extent to which its authority is engaged.

Why I Wrote This Book

The impetus for this treatise began during a dinner in the late 1990s with Fr. James Buckley, FSSP, when a discussion arose about the pro-life qualifications of a candidate for president of the United States. I claimed the candidate was pro-life, but Fr. Buckley in no small way disagreed. After about an hour of back and forth, Fr.

Buckley convinced me that the candidate was "selectively pro-life", meaning that the candidate opposed abortion, but with the usual three exceptions to his opposition: rape, incest, threat to the woman's life. Fr. Buckley's position was that the three exceptions disqualified him from claiming pro-life status because these exceptions assume that the intentional killing of an unborn child is not sinful when extenuating circumstances are present. He convinced me that induced abortion is an immoral medical procedure always, everywhere, and without exception. To be pro-life is to oppose induced abortion without exceptions.

The clincher in Fr. Buckley's argument was based on the distinction between moral and immoral medical procedures. Moral medical procedures are based on the intent to do good, to heal, to cure. Immoral medical procedures are based on misguided or evil intent. It is a fact that induced abortion intends to destroy the life of an unborn child, which is never a morally good intention. Thus, induced abortion is an obstetric procedure that should never be permitted.

CHAPTER 3

THE SCOPE OF THE PROTECTION OF THE UNBORN AND THE MESSAGE

Religious Significance of the Message

From a Catholic perspective, human life has a special dignity before God because God created human persons as body and soul with a purpose. No other creature in the known universe was created with the charge to be Godlike in the capacity of God's own image and likeness. Man is to have dominion over all of creation, from the earth out into space. He is to co-create human life with God. He is to live a life that is fully human, i.e., in accordance with his created nature. His primary moral commitment stems from his created nature: to know his God, love his God, and serve his God. His second moral commitment was summarized by Christ as "to love your neighbor as yourself" (Matthew 22:39). In as much as human life has a special dignity before God greater than that of all other earthly creatures, man has a special obligation to guard his neighbor's life as if it were his own (cf. Leviticus 19:16, NAB; Tanakh).

There are other works about the full scope of human dignity before God and man that explain why man is not free to take his own life, to cause the death of the elderly or infirm of mind or body, or to *unjustly* take the life of another man (cf. Pope Paul VI, 1965a). This treatise will not address these other moral concerns.

The present work endeavors only to explain why unjustly taking an unborn or recently-born human life is a grave moral evil always, everywhere, and for all time (Pope John Paul II, 1995).

Political Significance of the Message

The pro-life message today suffers from certain outdated definitions used universally by both those who defend life in the womb and those who discount its human value. Millions of voters in the United States do not favor the pro-life message because they: (1) received inadequate or no formal moral instruction in their school years, (2) have never been exposed to the rational arguments that favor the pro-life message, (3) have been confused by the disjointedness and contradictory nature of rhetoric by politicians that favor the pro-life message, (4) are confused about the proper moral object when a pregnant mother and her unborn child are under consideration, or (5) are convinced by obsolete terminology that the abortion proponents present a rational and ethical case. I believe that the continued use of outmoded terms has multiple causes, such as ignorance or inattentiveness to precision in the early definitions, and more recently in the ceding of the language of pregnancy to those who are in a certain sense trapped by their formal and clinical education, to others who entertain a notion of morality that diverges from the natural law, and to some who promote a political agenda at odds with right reason. Many have built their careers on acceptance of misleading terminology and do not give this acceptance a second thought. At the start of a re-specification of the common labels attached to certain medical procedures, it must be acknowledged that these labels have misled many people into thinking that the three exceptions generally written into pro-life laws are valid before God. In order to recommend a change in these labels, new labels must be devised. Support for this change is found in religion and reason. But since these categories of thinking are not deeply grasped by the average man in the pew, a dictionary of terms should accompany the argument for change. The dictionary of terms must include proper definitions of common words such as conscience, pregnancy, abortion, God, as well as more technical terminology such as medical condition, medical oath, human life, human person, legal person, true religion, and others. A more convincing explanation of the pro-life message can be offered once these terms are defined according to longstanding use—dating as far back as the ancient Greek philosophers and the first sources of divine revelation. A glossary of relevant terms is included at the end of this treatise.

The Legitimacy of Abortion?

Since the beginning of the 20th century, the answer to the question of the legitimacy of abortion has evolved from abortion being an unthinkable evil to abortion as a moral good to be embraced by all women. The confusion among many women is directly tied to confusion over the proper moral object in a pregnancy. The proper moral object in a pregnancy is twofold: protect the life of the mother *and* protect the life of the unborn child. Certain medical problems can cause the moral object to diverge from this simple scenario. There are situations where an illness or other medical problem can force a medical procedure where a healthy embryo is unintentionally removed from a mother's body in order to save the mother's life. Fortunately, the relative number of these situations is small. Unfortunately, medical science has not progressed sufficiently to enable these embryos to survive and develop outside of the womb. There are other situations where the growth of embryonic tissue can pose a risk to a woman's life, but this mass of tissue is not a living embryo. The more medically-complicated situations require special moral considerations, such as drawing upon the principle of double effect. Whenever the word "abortion" is used without adjectives in this treatise, it refers to "induced abortion". Induced abortion is always intentional.

Motives which determine the legitimacy of abortion in the minds of men are many and varied. Examples may include fear of parenthood, economic concerns, inconvenience of caring for a child, hatred of children or humanity in general, irreligion, and so on. In its most morally-defensible form, the question of the legitimacy of abortion in the modern age is not political or utilitarian, but religious. The choice of which religion to follow can be complicated by the type of government that exists where a person lives, availability of medical care, societal customs, family concerns, and other considerations. In accordance with *Dignitatis Humanae* (Pope Paul VI, 1965b), I consider the Catholic faith to be a true religion, a religion that must be followed if a person begins to recognize it as a true religion. But what makes a religion true in the eyes of God?

What Makes a Religion True?

A working definition of true religion might be the following: a set of beliefs inspired by God and a set of obligations demanded by God, which are necessary to hold and observe in order to be righteous before God. Catholics consider definitive the beliefs inspired by God and the obligations demanded by God which are found in the Catholic Bible and in the interpretations of these beliefs and demands as offered by the Magisterium. These beliefs and obligations were expounded and lived by Christ as personal guidance on how to be righteous before God. Judaism and Islam both have belief systems based in their own ways on the Old Testament, but they are religions that lack fulfillment and completion because they fail to recognize the dual nature of the God-man, Jesus Christ. Jesus Christ and His way are the fulfillment, completion, and perfection of the religion that followed in continuity from Adam through the Patriarchs, Abraham, Moses, and those who with sincerity followed the moral commitments in the law of Moses until the birth of Christ, (YouTube, 2025)

True religion presupposes an absolute standard of reality against which all moral and spiritual situations and realities are compared. In its simplest form, Christianity defines religion in its most fundamental terms as a discipline and lifestyle of doing and believing. The following are some examples from the New Testament:

> Religion that is pure and undefiled before God, the Father, is this: to care for orphans and widows in their affliction

> and to keep oneself unstained by the world. [James 1:27, *New Revised Standard Version*]

> …he that doth the will of my Father who is in heaven, he shall enter into the kingdom of heaven [Matthew 7:21, Rheims New Testament]

> But without faith it is impossible to please him, for anyone who approaches God must believe that he exists and that he rewards those who seek him. [Hebrews 11:6, NAB]

The highest act of religion in the Catholic Church is reception of the Eucharist. During reception of the Eucharist, the communicant offers his whole self to God, including his aspirations, fealty, thanksgiving, and praise. St. Paul in Romans 12:1 refers to this offering as a "reasonable service" or a "reasoned worship" (from the Greek: " λογικὴν λατρείαν ὑμῶν", the "reasonable service of you"). Accordingly, religion is viewed by Catholics as a reasonable service offered to God:

> I beseech you therefore, brethren, by the mercy of God, that you present your bodies a living sacrifice, holy, pleasing unto God, your reasonable service. [Rheims New Testament]

Numerous parallels to the "doing" aspect of religion are found in the Old Testament. Many examples are found in the *Decalogue* (the Ten Commandments) and in the *613 Commandments of Moses* (listed in Wikipedia). An Old Testament example of the need to believe is found in the book of Numbers, verse 14:11 (ERV, *English Revised Version*):

> And the LORD said unto Moses: "How long will this people despise Me? and how long will they not believe in Me, for all the signs which I have wrought among them?"

In some of the other major religions of the world, moral precepts that align with the Decalogue can be found as elements of true religion.

Some Practical Considerations

Elon Musk and other forward thinkers have figured out in the last few years that worldwide contraception and abortion may not be of benefit to the human race, after all. Even some eugenicists are jumping on board the "have more babies" train. An article a couple of years ago, titled "Meet the Elite Couples Breeding to Save Mankind", reported on an unintended consequence of the abortions of hundreds of millions of unborn infants around the world (Dodds, 2023):

> With global birth rates in free fall, Silicon Valley's "pronatalists" are aiming to halt the decline – by having as many babies as possible.

Another article a couple of days later went into greater detail (Mahdaw, 2023). This article is titled "'Hipster Eugenics': Why is the Media Cosying Up to People Who Want to Build a Super Race?" Here are some excerpts:

> The Collinses don't just want to increase the birth rate; they want to optimize the sort of children being born. They used genetic testing for their own embryos and, as Bloomberg reports, "created a spreadsheet with each embryo's scores, weighting them according to their desired mental health traits".
>
> ...Pro-natalism may mean pro-birth but the loudest voices in the movement are clearly only pro people like themselves being born. The most famous proponent was one Jeffrey Epstein, who planned to develop a super-race of humans with his DNA, by impregnating up to 20 women at a time. There is a constant refrain in pro-natal circles about how important it is for "really smart people" to keep reproducing.

Now these "pro-natalists" are not pro-life in any sense of the word. They are instead pro-self interest. They realize that declining populations can lead to problems for themselves and their offspring. Elon Musk observed the following (Porter, 2023):

> ..."[I]n the past we could rely upon...simple limbic system rewards in order to procreate. But once you have birth control and abortions and whatnot, now you can still satisfy limbic instinct, but not procreate."

> ..."I'm sort of worried that hey, civilization, if we don't make enough people to at least sustain our numbers, perhaps increase a little bit, then civilization's going to crumble."

Who benefits from children in families? The oldest generation in a family can benefit in old age by support from the younger generations as grandparents move beyond their most financially productive years. Society can benefit by the brainpower that new people can bring to every field of endeavor. The planet can benefit from new solutions to careless practices that can lead to increased pollution, ground and water contamination, possible changes to local and geographically larger climates, damage to ecosystems, and other human-induced problems in the natural environment. Families headed by a morally-grounded husband and wife can lead to a lower crime rate, happier neighborhoods and cities, sensible political structures, and global peace and tranquility.

But what about overpopulation, Malthusianism? If one's scope of existence is limited to life on planet earth, then an increasing population could plausibly stress "nonrenewable" resources. I place "nonrenewable" in quotation marks because human ingenuity can find ways to take advantage of existing resources in ways only dreamed of (or not even dreamed of) centuries earlier. Energy reaching the earth from the sun, energy reaching the earth's surface from below, energy produced by tidal forces in the sea, energy from the wind, energy from gravitational systems, energy from mineral deposits (such as hydrogen gas) trapped in sediments below the earth's surface; all sorts of energy sources are available right here on the earth. "Renewable" resources such as trees, rainfall, crops, fish, farm animals, and other resources have been and always are available for human use. Metallic resources from the ground can be recycled and used over and over again. Nonmetallic resources from the ground (sand, clay, lime, etc.) are in great abundance both on the surface and below it.

But what if Neo-Malthusianism is onto something, and humans could actually overuse the earth's natural mineral and water resources to the point of scarcity? Not to worry: God in His wisdom provided a solar system of planets, moons, and asteroids to satisfy our growing needs. Water, metals, natural gas, nonmetallic minerals, and other resources needed for human thriving are found throughout our solar system. In my studied opinion, the only thing lacking in the current technological age is the will to mine these resources. Instead of wasting exorbitant financial sums on the search to destroy God, i.e., the quest to find "life" on other planets, these expenditures would be better used in developing interplanetary ships to explore and mine the moons and asteroids in our solar system. Our own moon, Mars, and other solar system bodies could be colonized if the earth actually could become overpopulated. If suitable propulsion systems or other methods of traversing great distances in reasonable amounts of time were to be developed, interstellar travel might become a reality. This would open the entire galaxy to extraction of resources for human use. The totality of God's created universe, especially what we know about our solar system, suggests that it was designed to provide for life. The nature of matter, physical processes, biological systems and interactions, and consciousness are much better explained by design than by its opposite.

CHAPTER 4

ON LIFE

What is life?

One Secularist Perspective

According to some, life is nothing more than an organism consisting of solids, liquids, gases, biochemical reactions, and electrical impulses. This is considered the essence and substance of life. The nature of life is to subsist on our planet and enhance or detract from the planet's material purity. People, for example, are considered by some to be a blight on the planet, creatures that exist in a condition of exploiter and destroyer. People destroy forests; make animals go extinct; pollute air, ground, and water resources; exhaust and waste other natural resources; and prefer to kill one another rather than live in peace with each other and with nature. A dismal example of life.

Plants, on the other hand, are good. They produce oxygen, provide a sink for CO_2 and other undesirable gases, transfer water from the ground to the atmosphere to make rain, supply people with renewable resources, provide shade from the sun, and serve other beneficial purposes. A fine example of life.

Animals are mostly neutral. Some pose a threat to people, and when domesticated by man, they might even pose a threat to the planetary environment. Other than serving as nuisances, pets, or food sources, animals are basically a curiosity of nature.

One Religious Perspective

According to Catholicism, life is a good created by God to serve Him each in its own way. The majority of plants, animals, and most other things that find their home on or in our planet primarily serve God through their mere existence and functioning. Each creature of God (be it animate or inanimate) serves its Creator through its essence, substance, and nature. In elementary terms, the essence of a rock, for example, is to exist as a hard, lifeless, solid material of benefit in many ways to people. Its substance, in most basic terms, is to exist as an inanimate material being. Its nature is to serve as a support for mountains, buildings, roadways, altars, other constructions; as a decoration; as a tool or weapon; and for other human uses.

The essence of a man, on the other hand, was succinctly defined by Boethius (AD 520) as "an individual substance of a rational nature", i.e., a thinking being that exists as an individual person. Man exists in substance as a creature of body and soul (matter and spirit), with a nature capable of knowing, loving, and serving his Creator and his fellow man. His soul is said to be the form of his body. *Public revelation* informs us that man in his nature shares some of the attributes and abilities of his Creator, such as the ability to co-create human life, to steward our planet and any other celestial bodies that we many one day colonize, and to join together as husband and wife in a manner similar to God's union with mankind through Christ's Church. Man is not a blight on the earth as long as he decides to align his will with that of his Creator and to use creation in a way that best serves his Creator and his fellow creatures.

Is Life Important?

One Secularist Perspective

"Important" can be simply defined as "having relevant and crucial value" (Wiktionary). Imagine, if you will, a person who rejects belief in God, is a moral relativist, and does not believe in the Christian conception of an afterlife. I will refer to this person as an atheistic materialist. What is the relevant and crucial value of human life in the mind of an atheistic materialist? Just guessing here, but indications are that life has value to this person primarily from sentimental, utilitarian, and competitive perspectives. The sentimental aspect of life can realize an appreciation for family, friends, ancestors, pets, and possessions such as automobiles and houses. The importance of utility takes into consideration food, shelter, clothing, safety, and security. When these are provided for, contentment can ensue. The competitive aspect of "importance" is of equal magnitude as the other two because it bears on one's professional standing, social standing, comfort level (personal wealth), and pride in self, family, subordinates, and accomplishments. Greater meaning than these would be difficult to justify because the physicalist mindset of an atheistic materialist can discover only what the five senses can perceive—there is nothing transcendent to the material world, man, or mind.

One Religious Perspective

According to my understanding of Catholicism, life is important because God is its author. As the Author of creation, God has total command over the disposition of the universe and all that is contained within it. Since life is an important component of the universe, God's authority encompasses life's functioning and outcomes. Given, then, that God is "in control" of all aspects of creation, it is important that man recognize God's sovereignty over life and over man's relation to life. The concept of "in control", as used here, means that God sustains His creation, permits moral evils, and is the cause of physical goods and harms either directly or by His design of the principles ("laws") governing the universe. The reason why God permits moral evil is because He has endowed man with the freedom to choose to do good, even if man errs and chooses with his own free will to do evil. God always brings forth good from evil even if we do not always perceive the good that He has brought forth (D. Bouchard, personal communication, 15 August 2025).

Public revelation explains that man is so important to God that God cares about the eternal destiny of each human person, body and soul. This is the reason why God provided man with so many aids that he could live in such a way as to share in God's internal life while in this world (Pope John Paul II, 1995). God's standards for good moral behavior are known as God's justice. In Catholic terms, the virtue of justice inclines the will "to render to each and to all what belongs to them" (Slater, 1910). Attributes of justice and mercy are exercised in the here and now, and are likewise exercised at the time of transition from material life to purely spiritual life, i.e., at the moment of death, which is referred to by Catholics as the *particular judgment*. If God is so concerned about justice and mercy in the matter of the judgment of souls, then it stands to reason that men should be equally concerned with so important a reality. As bearing on the eternal reality, human life is therefore a temporal reality that ought to demand the greatest respect and attention of men.

If Life is Important, What About Death?

One Secularist Perspective

Death is the absolute end of life: a particular life ceases to exist at the death of this life. There is no "afterlife", no heaven, no hell, no consciousness or mental activity, no spiritual continuity of the human person after death. Death is an end to a meaningless existence. No God awaits the dead, only the inanimate earth and whatever creatures feed on the dead. To me, this is a depressing philosophy that leaves no room for joy.

Pascal's Wager

A contrary of this perspective was given by the French scientist and philosopher, Blaise Pascal. Short of a private revelation from

God, one of the best reasons why I would not bet my life on the atheistic-materialist perspective above was expressed by Pascal in a collection of notes published posthumously as "Pensées" (Pascal, 1670). In the briefest possible summary, Pascal's argument goes something like this. I should pattern my personal behavior and beliefs in such a way that a God of the Christians does exist. The reward in doing so is knowledge and happiness now and in the afterlife. But if there is no God of the Christians, then by patterning my life and belief system in the manner of a Christian, I lose nothing other than a few creature comforts and pleasures. This argument is called *Pascal's wager* and is considered rational by many.

One Religious Perspective

According to Catholicism, there is a God who cares about each of His creatures. This God is considered infinite in His many attributes, such as knowledge, wisdom, constancy, power, and others. As the creator of the universe, this God transcends the universe and exists in an essence known as the *Godhead*, a Godhead which consists of a unity of divine Persons. These Persons are distinguishable from one another solely on the basis of the relationship of one to the other. They are one and the same God in every other way that we can imagine. Sounds strange, but there are solid reasons for accepting a *mystery* such as this. This God who transcends nature is referred to as *supernatural.*

This God created the race of men to which we all belong. He created us with certain expectations about how we are to serve Him and each other. As the only unchanging Being in existence, the standards He sets for men are likewise unchanging. In their most primitive form, and as a basis for moral standards, these standards are summarized in divine revelation (Hebrews 11:6) as two-fold: to believe (1) that God exists, and (2) that He rewards those who seek him. The first of these standards is self explanatory, but the second could use some illumination. A reward can come about in several ways, but two of these will be cited here. The first is by *merit*, the second by *grace*. For this discussion, merit is defined as something worthy or deserving of reward. Grace is a free and undeserved assistance from God. In as much as a human being is a finite person with a definite beginning, the first reception of grace from God by a human person constitutes a life-altering event, even if the person is unaware that this grace has entered his soul. This first grace is offered by God to all men. It can be resisted, or it can be accepted. If accepted, the person is said to exist in a state of grace. For as long as the person remains in the state of grace, his moral actions can earn him merit before God if they are good. Grace is said to build upon grace, and likewise merit can build upon merit. Grace from God is supernatural and enables men to share in His divine life in a mysterious way, mysterious because our comprehension of this sharing is limited by our human intellect.

The sharing of the divine life of God in the temporal sphere (here and now) is a prelude to the sharing of this same life in the afterlife. Those who die while in this sharing relationship can continue and perfect this relationship with God in a condition referred to as *beatitude*. This condition is considered the highest good achievable by man with God's grace. This special beatitude is believed to continue for all eternity because human death transitions the person from the temporal sphere into the eternal sphere of existence. Eternal beatitude is the final τέλος (ultimate purpose) for which man was destined by God from the beginning. This is the reward for which Pascal wagers. Thus, the importance of death is its function as a portal to the afterlife.

Who Deserves to Live?

One Secularist Perspective

Those who can provide utility and happiness to their fellows are those who deserve to live. Thus, a newborn baby deserves to live because it can provide happiness to its family members and will potentially become a contributing member of society. The aged can deserve to live because they too can provide happiness to their family members and perhaps even an ongoing contribution to society. Similar reasoning can pertain to those who are disabled, injured, sick, or in other conditions considered less than ideal. All of these are theoretically protected from harm in the United States by the U.S. Constitution (especially the 14th Amendment), as illuminated in the preamble of the U.S. Declaration of Independence. Thus, all born persons who fall within the jurisdiction of U.S. law can be deserving of life and its preservation.

One Religious Perspective

One of the fundamental constituents of Catholic belief is that human life is a *gift* from God and because of this, God alone has sovereignty over life and death. However, as sharers in the life of the Godhead, God allows us to cooperate with His sovereignty in limited regulation of the affairs of men. For example, there are conditions under which one man is permitted by God to take the life of another man in self defense or defense of his neighbor's life. These conditions are defined by both moral and legal codes. With the exception of these conditions, all human persons deserve to live, regardless of their personal circumstances, including where they were born, their ancestry, and where they live.

The definition of a human person has always been clear going back into antiquity. There have been conjectures about the exact point of origin in time of a particular person's life, but there has been a consistent moral conviction among believers in the Christian God that depriving an unborn child the privilege of life is prohibited. Even certain Greeks, as shown in Chapter 2, acknowledged this. This prohibition is seen in the writings of the first Christians. Especially worthy of note is the 1st century Christian teaching known as the *Didache*, which says: "you shall not murder a child by abortion" (Kirby, 2023). If it can be established to a standard acceptable to all people who do not reject God that preborn human life has merit before God and man, then civil and criminal law should outlaw the direct taking of this life in all cases. According to the principle of double effect summarized in Chapter 2, there can be certain cases in which a preborn human life is lost due to medical complications during pregnancy. The loss of preborn life in these cases is indirect and unintentional. The first goal of this treatise is to simplify as much as possible the rationale behind the conviction that favors the life of the unborn child.

CHAPTER 5

A BRIEF NOTE ON THE NATURE OF SCIENCE AND THE DISTINCTION BETWEEN PHYSICAL AND BIOLOGICAL SCIENCE

Introduction

For those interested, in this chapter I will explain with discussion and examples my understanding of the nature of science, how practical science works, why science is important, and the relationship of science to God. I think this is useful because the specific purpose of this treatise is to serve as a proposal to redefine certain terms in medical science of relevance to unborn human life. Given that the natural sciences are normally divided between the biological and physical sciences, I think it important to briefly distinguish between the two on a basic level. After five decades of contemplating the relationship between religion and science, it is clear to me that the nature of the universe points to its governance by God.

The Contrast Between Religion and Science

In the context of religion, which makes the most sense: authority, revelation, reason? In Catholicism, all three are essential to understanding God and His interactions with men. Reason convinces that there must be a non-contingent First Cause, an entity that starts and may eventually bring to conclusion the universe He has created. Revelation fills in details that were either unknown or unable to be grasped without assistance from a higher intellect. Authority preserves the truth that is known, provides stability to what is now, and exercises wisdom in decisions about what may be new knowledge.

What about science? In the context of science, which makes the most sense: authority, reason, or revelation? In science, reason, as the first interpreter of experimental results, ought to take priority, but in practice, authority plays a major role in decision-making. The authority of precedent, empirical demonstration, and the wisdom of experience—the experience of one man or of many—these are qualities that give heft to authority. Does revelation have any role in science? Many scientists, especially experimental scientists, discover through their work that order, predictability, and ultimate non-contingency reveal a power greater than the physical universe. Thus, many acknowledge the reality of God and trust that even if their own experimental results can seem mysterious to them, they are known to the One who is responsible: (1) for all that is, (2) for every action that can possibly take place, and (3) for light at the ultimate end of the tunnel.

Brief Note About the Sciences and Engineering

Unlike religion, the natural sciences (e.g., physics, geology, biology, chemistry) are strictly concerned only with the material world. Science uses the five senses to learn, understand, and put to good use that which is physical in nature. Science observes nature and the products of human endeavor and produces hypotheses, theories, and paradigms to explain what is observed or expected. Science compares observations and measurements to relevant standards in order to determine the success or failure of its hypotheses, theories, and paradigms. Many of these standards are dependent on human perception, others on physical realities that can be known with certainty, others as the results of the logic of induction and deduction. There are other "standards" created by the mind of man that may not: (1) align with physical reality, (2) be testable, (3) be predictive, or (4) in other ways be useful to the human condition. These are known as opinions which can be either true or false. One of the greatest values of science, beyond the knowledge it provides of the natural world, is its ability to predict what can or will happen under well-defined circumstances. Whereas the results of engineering science are assessed by whether its products function in accordance with their design specifications, the predictions of natural science can be more open ended. Revisions to the predictions of natural science are often needed because nature is not always easy to comprehend and our understanding of its processes and properties generally increases with time.

On the Physical and Biological Sciences

Take the theory of plate tectonics as an example of an application of the physical sciences. Plate tectonics is a modern paradigm in the physical sciences that answers questions with a testable certitude that exceeds previous attempts to explain the "how" of solid-earth processes and events. Plate tectonics has solid predictive strength based on our understanding of the mechanisms acting in the earth's interior. Plate tectonics assists in the prediction of earth surface interactions such as earthquakes, volcanic eruptions, and landslides, but usually within the framework of regional probabilities within specified time windows. The theory of biological evolution is another example. It attempts to explain the natural origin and changes in lifeforms from the geologic past into the present. The theory can be divided into *macroevolution* (changes at the level of *species*) and *microevolution* (small-scale changes within species that are easily observable). The theory of macroevolution (actually a consensus paradigm) cannot, however, offer the same predictive strength as plate tectonics because it is a theory that is viewed as more highly probabilistic than the more deterministic physical theory (Blount, 2018; Mas, 2020). It is a theory that at the level of complex lifeforms looks backward, rather than forward (Luckow, 1995). Chance events at the molecular level and at the population level are thought to build upon one another to produce an increase in complexity in lifeforms under the assumption that vast numbers of events by trial and error must result in increases in complexity.

Maybe it is because I have more training, experience, and faith in the physical sciences than I have in theoretical biology that I have trouble believing that chance occurrences can lead to an increase in complexity in living things. This certainly does not happen in the earth's atmosphere. Take atmospheric turbulence as an example. Turbulence is a theory and a process described by statistics, "universal" laws, asymptotes, and the results of advanced dimensional analysis. It is the nearest phenomenon that I know of to unpredictability when viewed from minute to minute. Yet the random-style fluctuations in turbulent flows (Liau, 2025) never lead to an increase in complexity or order. Can biological systems, in the absence of intervention from outside, actually become more complex because of chance interactions of molecules and populations? I fail to see how this is rationally possible. In other words, every complexity created by man, be it a work of art, a building, an airplane, or crossbreeding of horses, requires the creativity of a human mind. These creations are not the product of random thinking or daydreaming, but rather they originate in a design produced in an ordered human intellect. According to true religion, the entire universe and everything in it, including processes, originated in the mind of God according to His design. Thus, even processes that appear mysterious (e.g., possessing random qualities) are known and created by God according to His plan.

Is it possible that biological evolution is a creation of God, based on a design that is exceedingly difficult for modern man to understand? Even though what I remember from my historical geology, marine science, and biology courses from five decades ago is now partially obsolete, there is still validity in the basics. Biological evolution can be defined as changes in physical or behavioral characteristics of biological populations that are passed on from parents to offspring over successive generations (cf. National Academy of Sciences, 2025). This definition says nothing about design, purpose, or progress. It merely says "change". The first level of evolutionary change is molecular—the *mutation*. Mutations occur as changes in a *DNA* molecule. DNA (deoxyribonucleic acid) is a large molecule that carries genetic information for the development and functioning of an organism (Bates, 2025). The DNA molecule can replicate into an identical DNA molecule. An error can happen during replication which damages the molecule. The molecule can also be damaged by other causes, such as chemicals, high-energy radiation, or environmental factors like extreme temperatures (Chatterjee, 2017). After DNA is damaged, damage-response mechanisms begin to repair the damage. If the repaired DNA is changed from the original molecule, it is called a mutation. According to an article about the constancy and uniformity of mutations over time, the authors note that mutations have random qualities, and their occurrence is understood as mathematically probable, not physically deterministic (Fitzgerald, 2019).

Being undesigned and purposeless, according to the consensus biological opinion, differences in genomes (genetic information) among different species which might suggest that one species found its origin in another should not be taken to indicate any sort of advancement or progression in value. According to this perspective, human beings, although more complex in composition and enhanced in capabilities, are no more special than bacteria. This perspective asserts that there is no created, spiritual human soul. There is only one species competing for survival against another. Should human beings one day destroy each other completely by technological means (e.g., war, pollutants or contaminants, biological agents), the bacteria will have proven themselves superior to us, since they will remain, while we went extinct. From the standpoint of a human person, this is not a very optimistic outlook for the future. The philosophy behind the conjecture of undesigned and purposeless is sterile, i.e., it holds no room for God and must therefore be rejected by one who believes and practices true religion.

I would like to comment on how sure we are about forecasts made by the physical sciences. My technical fields of training and experience are primarily in geophysical sciences, radiological physics, sensor development, and radar engineering. The following observations are in the area of geophysical sciences. Plate tectonics is a solid paradigm for understanding the basic physics of earth movements, forces in the earth system, and processes that cause earthquakes, volcanic eruptions, tsunamis, mountain building, and earth surface features. Yet we can only forecast the timing and location of earthquakes and volcanic eruptions as likelihoods within certain time windows and geographic regions. Astronomy and astrophysics have developed a workable understanding of planetary motions around a star and reasonable speculations about the interiors of the sun, planets, and moons in our solar system; made observations of the physical fields (e.g., electrical, magnetic, gravitational) between the celestial bodies in our solar system; and made observations of the type of matter that occupies the space between the planets and our sun. Yet we were taken off guard by the realization that the solar system has water molecules nearly everywhere, when until these recent discoveries were made it was believed that the solar system, apart from the earth, was a very dry place (Russell, 2017). Meteorology understands the basics of the physics and dynamics of the earth's atmosphere and its interactions with solar wind, the ground surface, and water bodies. Yet weather forecasts from day to day, but certainly not more than two or three days in advance, are offered in terms of regional probabilities instead of exact times and places where weather events such as rainfall and tornadoes will occur. When climate modeling results are compared to observed global temperature trends dating from when the models were first developed, what had been seen a few years ago was a notable overestimation of temperatures by the majority of models when compared to both satellite and reliable surface temperature measurements (Spencer, 2014; Mandock, 2014). I do not know if the models have improved since then.

Turning to the biological sciences, consider the inability of biological evolution to predict the next stage in "advancement" of breathing lifeforms, advancement being defined as an increase in complexity or perhaps physical or mental ability. The most the evolution paradigm can tell us is that "change" will take place and that this change depends on the environment in which these creatures live, the interactions between one species and another, bacterial and viral infections, and other "evolutionary pressures" that may be acting on them. According to the paradigm, the transitions between higher-order species (macroevolution) are speculated (i.e., not reproducible or observable in real time), the reasons for the transitions are contingent on chance events, and future advancements in complexity cannot be predicted.

What distinguishes forecasts made by the physical sciences from the speculations of macroevolution is that in every earthquake, volcanic, weather, and climate forecast, we know the nature of the outcome that we expect; it is basically only a matter of time before a predictable event occurs. This is not the case for macroevolution. The nature of "change" in macroevolution is so unconstrained that it cannot be predicted. Only "change" itself is postulated.

As a concrete example, compare the evolutionary process of undirected change to the well-understood deterministic phenomenon of "isostatic rebound". During the last Ice Age, the weight of ice sheets around the world exerted a downward pressure on the earth's crust below. As the ice sheets later melted during climate warming, the overlying weight was removed, and the crust began to rise in elevation relative to sea level. The rise is measurable, the reason for it is deterministic, and future rising can be predicted. The physical process is called isostatic rebound and is produced by rheological buoyancy. According to plate tectonics, the crust and rigid upper mantle behave as a unit called the lithosphere and overlie a more deformable zone in the upper mantle. As ice accumulates on the surface of the crust during an ice age, the additional weight of the ice forces the lithosphere downward, and the mantle below deforms or flows away from the overloaded region. During periods of global warming, the glacial ice melts, and the removal of ice by melting allows the lithosphere below to rise buoyantly as the deformable zone recovers.

Another well-known phenomenon in solid-earth geophysics is "delamination", a process whereby part of the lithosphere beneath the crust "peels off" from the remainder above. This process can predict, for example, the ongoing isostatic rise of the Appalachian Mountains, a rise that is slowed by erosion (Mandock, 2016). Geological delamination is predictable, but difficult to observe.

As noted above, the greater value of predictability in the physical sciences than in macroevolution is that physical sciences can predict quite precisely the outcomes of physical processes that are well-understood, such as the falling of a raindrop, whereas macro-evolution can postulate only "change". On the other hand, it has been clear for centuries that microevolution takes place in nature. Although microevolutionary changes may be variations in a complexity that already exists, they are not to be viewed as increases in complexity that must lead to "higher" forms of life. On the level of human intervention, selective breeding and the results of medical research can be beneficial to man and animal. These are engineered changes and advancements guided by human ingenuity. Although selective breeding and certain forms of medical research produce results like those of microevolution, these practices are directed and purposeful. The only way that I can see "nature" or "the universe" engineering macroevolutionary advancements in complexity is if a force that transcends nature and the universe is causing the advancements. Catholics would call this force the personal God of Christianity.

St. Augustine's Warning

In the 19th chapter of St. Augustine's first book on his allegorical interpretation of the first three chapters of the biblical book of Genesis, he offers a detailed warning about the danger of interpreting the Bible as if it were a science textbook. (Augustine of Hippo, 415). He points out that even the unlettered know something about the physical world, such as the movements of the planets, the seasons of the year, the eclipses of the sun and moon, the difference between plants and animals, the difference between the states of matter, and so forth. This knowledge can be learned from reason and experience. Now if a Christian teacher were to speak nonsense on these topics, not only would he show his ignorance and be judged foolish, but non-Christians might think that the writers of Scripture held such erroneous opinions. How could a non-Christian person familiar with basic scientific facts take seriously any attempt at the teaching of religion by a Christian who is ignorant of the type of common knowledge of the physical world that is gleaned from experience and the light of reason?

CHAPTER 6

ON THE CONJUGAL EMBRACE AND THE ORIGIN AND NATURE OF MAN

Male and Female He Created Them

One Secularist Perspective

This section is restricted to animals and people that reproduce in a manner like that of a man and a woman who are married to one another. Dogs copulate, cats copulate, cows copulate, people unmarried to one another copulate. Dogs "have sex", cats "have sex", cows "have sex", people unmarried to one another "have sex". The verb form of the word "sex", the equivalent of copulation, represents biological acts involving male and female reproductive organs. Any species with suitable plumbing can "have sex". "Having sex" is instinctual.

Where did "having sex" come from? By the consensus of those who have "earned the right to have a voice", "having sex" evolved as a preferred mechanism to populate species. Given the pragmatic moral neutrality of "having sex", no one has to be married to do it. Just find a suitable "partner", and have at it. No guilt. No serious consequences in secular culture. Contraception and abortion are available as needed. Sort of reminds me of the asinine advice offered by a certain high-level U.S. government official when he was asked in early 2020 if a person should be concerned by what might become a Covid pandemic. As I recall, his advice was to go to Italy, find a girl, and go to the beach.

Some Religious Perspectives

To understand the nature of the *conjugal embrace*, we must first understand the origin and nature of man. Just as all creatures owe their existence to God, all actions owe their origin to God's design for the universe and all that it contains. This is the Christian perspective. One of the attributes of God is omnipotence: He designed the universe, created the universe, maintains the universe, and will eventually allow the universe, as we know it, to end. Another of His attributes is omniscience. God knows His creation. Although finite intellects, such as man's, are unable to comprehend in a deterministic manner certain observations in nature such as unexpected quantum phenomena and turbulence in fluids, God has no such limitations. What appears random or even chaotic to man is deterministic (cause and effect) to God. He created the universe and allowed all the results that are believed to have stemmed from His creation. These results are described by modern science according to physical and biological theories.

But in addition to creating and working through natural causes, God can effect supernatural events. These supernatural events we call *miracles*. If biological evolution is a valid attempt to explain the diversity of species in the geologic record and today, then who is to say that the conditions needed for the diversity of lifeforms to evolve were not created by God? For example, the *Goldilocks hypothesis* suggests that for a planet to be hospitable to human life, it must meet a list of criteria (Tarbuck, 2012). The planet must: (1) be the right size, (2) be geologically active according to the plate tectonics model, (3) have a molten metallic core that generates a strong magnetic field, (4) be the right distance from its sun and other planets, (5) allow the buildup of an oxygen atmosphere at the right time after its formation, (6) be subject to asteroid impacts and massive volcanism at the right times in its geologic history, (7) orbit the right *size* star, (8) orbit the right *type* of star that produces a heliosphere capable of protecting the planet from cosmic rays. Are we just lucky to have all these criteria fall into place at the right time, or is a higher power actually involved?

If God exists according to the Christian understanding, then can He not be allowed to create as He sees fit? In other words, is He too weak to have designed the earth in such a way that allows for the appearance and disappearance of distinct lifeforms found in the fossil record? Is He not allowed to create any given species as He sees fit? Is He not allowed to create man as poetically described in the biblical book of Genesis?

St. Augustine in his *De Genesi ad Literam*, St. Basil in his *Hexameron*, and St. Thomas Aquinas in his *Summa Theologiae* all acknowledge in their own way that Chapter 1 of Genesis describes a process that does not substantively conflict with *one* of the *philosophical underpinnings* of the consensus view on biological evolution. In both the Genesis account of God's creative work and the consensus view of biological evolution, various lifeforms on the earth arose from the earth: in the one account, forms of life arose by creative acts of the Creator God, and in the other account, forms of life arose according to speculation based on an evolutionary paradigm that extends from ancient times until today. Augustine, Basil, and Aquinas point out that early in earth history God created the material world in such a way that the earth could "bring forth" by His hand certain variations of lifeforms. Unless otherwise noted, all the Scriptural quotations in this section are taken from the Douay Old Testament (Challoner revision). From verses 11-24 of Genesis 1:

> Let the earth bring forth the green herb, and such as may seed, and the fruit tree yielding fruit after its kind, which may have seed in itself upon the earth. ...Let the waters bring forth the creeping creature having life, and the fowl that may fly over the earth under the firmament of heaven. ...Let the earth bring forth the living creature in its kind, cattle and creeping things, and beasts of the earth, according to their kinds.

Throughout the history of Christianity, allegorical interpretations of Scripture have accompanied the literal interpretations. Literal interpretations of the origin of the universe usually begin with 6 physical days of creation, with each day being 24 hours in duration. This interpretation cannot be definitively ruled out, since no man was around to either confirm or deny these 6 days. However, several of the Church fathers sought ways to interpret Genesis 1 in ways that would not conflict with the findings of natural science. St. Augustine's warning comes to mind. One allegorical interpretation redefines the understanding of "let there be light" (Genesis 1:3). Instead of physical light, St. Augustine's allegorical interpretation says the light was the light of angelic intellect. During the six days of creation, he envisions morning to be God revealing his step-by-step plan to the angels and night as the angels contemplating what they had just received: 6 revelations, corresponding to 6 "days". Augustine also reinterprets the "days" of creation to be merely a sequence that was offered "together", or at the same time ("simul", in Ecclesiasticus 18:1): 6 revelations, each distinguished from one another by a different place in the sequence of revealing. There was no time interval of a 24-hour day between each successive revelation; all 6 were revealed together, but the angelic intellect needed to sequence them to contemplate each one individually.

Another allegorical interpretation of the six days of creation in Genesis 1 (Aquinas, 1274) offers an outline of two parallel sequences of events, each sequence having a rough chronological ordering that follows (with one glaring exception) the consensus theorized by science of the evolution of the universe and life on earth. According to this allegorical interpretation, the first three days of creation outline a sequence that can be thought of as the creation of structures or "distinctions", and the second three days can be considered "adornments" (or content) of these structures. Astrophysical science describes the evolution of the universe as an expansion from a single point into what exists today. The dominant paradigm underlying astrophysics is referred to as the *Big Bang* theory. Biological science clings to the evolutionary paradigm described in Chapter 5. Just as astrophysics does not know what existed before the Big Bang, biological evolution does not know how life is supposed to have arisen from inanimate matter without intervention from God. There are imaginative hypotheses, but nothing observable in real time or reproducible.

In the biblical creation sequence, there was no universe (material world) before God created light (energy): there was only "void and empty".

> In the beginning God created heaven, and earth. And the earth was void and empty, and darkness was upon the face of the deep; and the spirit of God moved over the waters. [Genesis 1:1-2]

In these verses, "heaven and earth" can be taken as referring to all that exists in creation. "Void and empty" suggest that God created *ex nihilo*: from nothing into something. As far as the Big Bang model is concerned, "void and empty" is a good way to describe existence before the universe was born. According to this model, material existence (the universe) began with energy expanding outward into the void and emptiness from the point of origin.

On the first day of the "distinction" sequence of the biblical creation account, God made light (Genesis 1:3), which is a form of energy. After God made light, He "divided the light from the darkness" (Genesis 1:4). The darkness typically represents "void and empty", or it allegorically might represent matter. According to the Big Bang theory, during the expansion of the early universe, matter formed, and photon radiation (think of it as light) decoupled (separated) from the matter: light and matter separated from one another.

On the second day in the "distinction" creation sequence, creation began to take on order (Genesis 1:6-8). In the Big Bang model, after the light separated from the matter, the universe began to take on order.

On the third day in the "distinction" creation sequence, the ordering of the earth into land and sea began, and plants were "brought forth". According to historical geology, after the earth formed, continents and seas formed. After the formation of land and sea, in a certain sense the precursors to plant life formed. According to historical geology, cyanobacteria are thought to be among the earliest forms of life in the fossil record, and they might be considered precursors to plant life because they produce oxygen through photosynthesis. These plant precursors are believed to be older than more complex lifeforms, such as plants, fish, reptiles, birds ("feathered dinosaurs"), and other animals, because they appear lower in the stratigraphic sequencing of the fossil record than the more complex lifeforms.

The sequence of adornments follows the sequence of structures or "distinctions". The sequence of adornments stands on its own chronology in terms of proper sequencing but does not follow the sequence of "distinctions" without interruption. The interruption occurs with the first day of adornments (fourth day in the biblical creation account) preceding the last day of "distinctions" (third day in the biblical creation account), as matter was being organized and ordered. The creation of the solar system and stars represents this ordering, and their purpose was to be adornments of (i.e., adding content to) the universe. The fifth day came after the third and fourth days, and with it the adornment of the sea and sky through the "bringing forth" on the earth of fish, reptiles, and birds (the first birds being categorized by paleontology as flying reptiles). The sixth day followed the fifth, and on this day the earth was adorned with animals and finally man. I have summarized these sequences for greater clarity in the table below.

Conventional Science	**First 3 Days of Creation (Distinction)**	**Last 3 Days of Creation (Adornment)**
The Beginning Energy expanded from the point of origin into the emptiness.	**Day 1** God made light (a form of energy). He then separated the light from the darkness (the "void and empty").	**Day 4** God created the solar system and stars to adorn the universe He had just created.
Organization & Ordering Normal matter formed from the cooling of hot plasma. Photon radiation decoupled from the normal matter. Gravity condensed clouds of hydrogen into stars & galaxies.	**Day 2** God created matter and began to organize and order it.	**Day 5** God adorned the earth's sea and sky through the appearance of fish, reptiles, and birds.
The Earth Internal earth processes and plate tectonics created low-density land masses that rose above sea level. Photosynthetic	**Day 3** God organized the earth into land and sea. God created the first plants.	**Day 6** God adorned the earth with animals and finally man.

bacteria appear near the bottom of rock strata sequencing. More complex lifeforms appear higher in this sequencing.		

Bergsma and Pitre introduce their own allegory in their biblical introduction and commentary by relating the parallel sequences of structure and adornment to a "liturgical orientation of creation" (Bergsma, 2018). In their interpretation, instead of Genesis 1:2 being translated as "void and empty", it can be translated as "without form and empty". According to their interpretation, the first sequence (first three days of creation) addresses the first privation of creation ("without form") by providing structure, while the second sequence (the last three days of creation) addresses the second privation ("empty") by providing content. The "distinctions" of the first three days are the structures of creation, and the adornments of the last three days are the content of these structures.

Having briefly introduced some outline interpretations (scientific and religious) of the origin of the universe, the earth, and life on the earth, I would like to now focus on the origin of man. Consider that even though the modern scientific consensus eschews the Christian religion and considers man to be just another product of evolutionary diversity, God is not bound by any human consensus opinion. Consider verses 26-28 from Genesis 1:

> And he said: Let us make man to our image and likeness: and let him have dominion over the fishes of the sea, and the fowls of the air, and the beasts, and the whole earth, and

> every creeping creature that moveth upon the earth. And God created man to his own image: to the image of God he created him: male and female he created them. And God blessed them, saying: increase and multiply, and fill the earth, and subdue it, and rule over the fishes of the sea, and the fowls of the air, and all living creatures that move upon the earth.

If there is any literal truth in these verses, then man may indeed have found his origin in a distinctly different event from the evolutionary construct. Consider verse 7 of Genesis 2:

> And then the Lord God formed man from the clay of the earth, and he breathed into his face the breath of life, and man became a living soul. [Catholic Public Domain Version]

It is possible that macroevolution, if directed by God's wisdom and power, might have brought a beast to the threshold of becoming a man, but it is also possible that man was created in a separate act directly from existing matter. In either case, what distinguishes a man from a beast is man's immortal soul, interpreted from this verse as "the breath of life". Given the complexity of animal organs and life processes, especially in the human person, it would require more faith for me to believe in macroevolution without God than I have in true religion and the Christian God.

Did the first woman evolve independently of the first man? I doubt this is likely, given the time scales of macroevolution and the lifetime of men. Did God breathe a soul into the woman's body at the same point in her creation that He did for the man? Science has nothing to say about this, but Genesis does. Verses 21-22 of Genesis 2:

> Then the Lord God cast a deep sleep upon Adam: and when he was fast asleep, he took one of his ribs, and filled up flesh for it. And the Lord God built the rib which he took from Adam into a woman: and brought her to Adam.

Transhuman, you say? A step upward in human evolution? Doubtful, given that women are as truly human as men are. Even though the description for creation of the woman comes across as a bit more poetic than the one for creation of the man, the point of the Genesis account is driven home in the verse that follows:

> And Adam said: This now is bone of my bones, and flesh of my flesh; she shall be called woman, because she was taken out of man. [Genesis 2:23]

The next verse reveals the first-ever conjugal embrace:

> Wherefore a man shall leave father and mother, and shall cleave to his wife: and they shall be two in one flesh. [Genesis 2:24]

Is the act of Adam cleaving to his wife and becoming "one flesh" with her an example of "having sex"? Of mere copulation? It is not. Why? Because Eve is blessed by God as Adam's legitimate wife. The sacred covenant of matrimony between a man and his wife before God raises the physical joining to include a spiritual embrace. The sexual act between Adam and Eve is no longer "just physical", but both physical and spiritual. Catholic theology refers to the act as the conjugal embrace. Besides unification of the spouses, the conjugal embrace is open to producing a new life within a family. This marital act is not only open to conceiving a new life, but is predicated on an embrace by the husband, wife, and other family members of the new life both *before* and *after* birth. Children are a creation of God to be nurtured and raised by a husband and wife in the community of the family.

We saw in the Genesis verses above that God infused a soul into the man, and to make the woman fully human, we reason that He likewise breathed a soul into her as well. It is reasonable to assume that the soul was infused into the man immediately on his being created (cf. Pope Pius XII, 1950). It is also reasonable to conclude that the same happened for Eve, in as much as she was to have an equal share in humanity as the man. This immediacy of infusion of a soul into Adam and into Eve is found to have repercussions later in this treatise.

CHAPTER 7

ON IN VITRO FERTILIZATION, CONTRACEPTION, AND NATURAL FAMILY PLANNING

What's Wrong With In Vitro Fertilization and Contraception

Catholicism believes the purpose of the conjugal embrace to be twofold: (1) the unity of the spouses, male and female; (2) the co-creation of human life with God. Unless otherwise noted, all Scriptural quotations in this chapter are taken from the Douay Old Testament and the Rheims New Testament (Challoner revision of each). The unification of one male and one female as husband and wife is one of the first commandments issued by God (Genesis 2:24) to the first human beings:

> Wherefore a man shall leave father and mother, and shall cleave to his wife: and they shall be two in one flesh.

Christ expounds (Matthew 19:3-6) on this unification:

> And there came to him the Pharisees tempting him, saying: Is it lawful for a man to put away his wife for every cause? Who answering, said to them: Have ye not read, that he who made man from the beginning, made them male and female? And he said: For this cause shall a man leave father

> and mother, and shall cleave to his wife, and they two shall be in one flesh. Therefore now they are not two, but one flesh. What therefore God hath joined together, let no man put asunder.

On revisiting Genesis 1:27-28, one can see another of the first commandments—that command about the second purpose of the conjugal embrace: to bear children.

> And God created man to his own image: to the image of God he created him: male and female he created them. And God blessed them, saying: Increase and multiply, and fill the earth, and subdue it, and rule over the fishes of the sea, and the fowls of the air, and all living creatures that move upon the earth.

Genesis 4:1-2 shows that this command was carried out by our first parents:

> And Adam knew Eve his wife; who conceived and brought forth Cain, saying: I have gotten a man through God. And again she brought forth his brother Abel.

The importance of this dual principle in Catholicism cannot be overstated, for it is on the basis of this principle that Catholic teaching about *artificial human procreation* and *contraception* can be understood. Whereas *in vitro* fertilization (a method of artificial human procreation where a human egg is fertilized outside of a female's body), *in vivo* fertilization (also known as artificial insemination, a method of artificial human procreation where a human egg is fertilized inside a female's body), and *embryo transfer* (abbreviated "ET", another method of artificial human procreation where a human embryo is placed in the uterus of a human female) frustrate the first purpose of the conjugal embrace (i.e., the physical joining of the husband and wife), contraception frustrates the second (i.e., the co-creation of a human life). Excerpts from *Donum Vitae*, an instruction on respect for human life as it originates and on procreation, explain the problems with these procedures (Sacred Congregation for the Doctrine of the Faith, 1987):

> Introduction
>
> 4. The fundamental values connected with the techniques of artificial human procreation are two: the life of the human being called into existence and the special nature of the transmission of human life in [matrimony]. The moral judgment on such methods of artificial procreation must therefore be formulated in reference to these values…
>
> 5. …From the moment of conception, the life of every human being is to be respected in an absolute way because…from its beginning [human life] involves "the creative action of God" and it remains forever in a special relationship with the Creator, who is its sole end. God alone is the Lord of life from its beginning until its end: no one can, in any circumstance, claim for himself the right to destroy directly an innocent human being. Human procreation re-

> quires on the part of the spouses responsible collaboration with the fruitful love of God; the gift of human life must be actualized in [matrimony] through the specific and exclusive acts of husband and wife...
>
> II. Interventions Upon Human Procreation
>
> 4.a. The Church's teaching on marriage and human procreation affirms the "inseparable connection, willed by God and unable to be broken by man on his own initiative, between the two meanings of the conjugal act: the unitive meaning and the procreative meaning. Indeed, by its intimate structure, the conjugal act, while most closely uniting husband and wife, makes them capable of the generation of new lives, according to laws inscribed in the very being of man and of woman"...
>
> ...Contraception deliberately deprives the conjugal act of its openness to procreation and in this way brings about a voluntary dissociation of the ends of [matrimony]...
>
> ...fertilization is licitly sought when it is the result of a "conjugal act which is per se suitable for the generation of children to which [matrimony] is ordered by its nature and by which the spouses become one flesh"...

There are other moral problems with artificial human procreation beyond first principles. Bishop Michael Burbridge explains these problems in a 2025 pastoral letter that specifically addresses in vitro fertilization (IVF). Below is a summary of the moral concerns he raises in this letter, which are direct quotations (Burbridge, 2025).

> …many of the embryonic children brought about by the process will either be discarded, having been deemed undesirable, or frozen, having been deemed desirable but unnecessary…
>
> …All children conceived and born through IVF possess inalienable human dignity. Indeed, their innate dignity is the reason for the Church's opposition to their being instrumentalized and made into objects by means of IVF, which eugenically selects some to live and others to die.
>
> …such procedures in fact replace rather than assist the loving self-gift of spouses manifest in procreative and unitive marital love. In this way, the natural and loving embrace of man and woman expressed in marital love is effectively replaced by a laboratory procedure made possible by the subjugation of man and woman to a technological process…
>
> …Unlike the adoption process, which has historically involved many safeguards and standards to ensure that adoptees are brought into a loving and stable family, IVF allows for virtually any single individual or unmarried couple, including those practicing lifestyles at odds with family happiness and stability, to obtain a child either directly or by means of an often economically vulnerable surrogate…
>
> …all children "have a right to be born to their married mother and father, through a personal act of self-giving

> love. IVF, however well-intended, breaches this bond and these rights and, instead, treats human beings like products or property. This is all the more true in situations involving anonymous donors or surrogacy"...
>
> ...A federal IVF entitlement or mandate would represent...an illegitimate handing over to Caesar the things of God (cf. Mk. 12:17)—the gift of human life and the good of the family from which society springs—would involve serious injustices, and over time would invite abuse, domination, and even subjugation to the raw power of the state. ...such a state mandate would inevitably result in the widespread coercion of healthcare workers and the evisceration of their professional right of conscience.

Donum Vitae explains the true identity of every human embryo, including those resulting from artificial methods of human procreation (Sacred Congregation for the Doctrine of the Faith, 1987):

> Although the manner in which human conception is achieved with IVF and ET cannot be approved, every child which comes into the world must in any case be accepted as a living gift of the divine Goodness and must be brought up with love.
>
> ...This doctrinal reminder provides the fundamental criterion for the solution of the various problems posed by the development of the biomedical sciences in this field: since

> the embryo must be treated as a person, it must also be defended in its integrity, tended and cared for, to the extent possible, in the same way as any other human being as far as medical assistance is concerned.

The United States Conference of Catholic Bishops (USCCB) has updated with revised commentary and definitions its summary guidelines for the use of reproductive technologies by Catholic married couples (Klaus, 2025). The guidelines are specific, instructive, and inclusive of highly detailed definitions.

How to Refer to the Destruction of Nascent Human Life

I remind the reader that I am not a medical professional, philosopher, or bioethicist. I cite only those sources that I believe necessary to frame in a Catholic perspective arguments and definitions that I will propose. In accordance with my understanding of Catholic teaching and of common belief, I propose to define abortion in this treatise specifically as *the direct termination of a pregnancy, from conception to birth, with the intent to destroy a human life*. This definition of abortion is often preceded by terms such as "induced", "direct", or "procured", as can be seen, for example, in the definition for an "induced termination of pregnancy" in the state of Georgia: "the purposeful interruption of pregnancy with the intention other than to produce a live-born infant or to remove a dead fetus and which does not result in a live birth" (GA Code § 31-10-1 (2024)). I cite this definition because Georgia is my state of residency in the U.S.

I also propose to define pregnancy in this treatise as *the condition of carrying developing offspring within a woman's body*. The definition aligns with definitions found in four U.S. major medical dictionaries (Gacek, 2009). As cited in Gacek, Dorland's *American Illustrated Medical Dictionary* pre-1950 definition of pregnancy was: "the condition of being with child". Dorland's definition beginning in 1951 and continuing at least through 2006 is: "the condition of having a developing embryo or fetus in the body, after union of an ovum and spermatozoon". The definition, as cited in Gacek, found in the 2006 edition of Mosby's medical dictionary is: "the gestational process, comprising the growth and development within a woman of a new individual from conception through the embryonic and fetal periods to birth". As cited in Gacek, the definition found in the editions of Stedman's medical dictionary from 1912-1995 was: "the state of a female after conception until the birth of the child". *Taber's Cyclopedic Medical Dictionary*, as cited in Gacek, had this definition from 1940-1970: "the condition of being with child". However, this dictionary changed its definition in the 2005 edition: "the condition of having a developing embryo or fetus in the body, after successful conception".

It is important to define the terms "abortion" and "pregnancy" in this treatise because of the many and varied notions applied to their meaning. As seen elsewhere in this chapter, these definitions do not contradict the usage by the Catholic Church.

Given the definitions above, is it proper to refer to the killing of human embryos outside of a woman's body as abortion? Pope John Paul II (1995) in his encyclical *Evangelium Vitae* distinguishes between the killing of in vitro embryos and direct abortion (emphases mine):

> ...direct abortion, that is, abortion willed as an end or as a means, always constitutes a grave moral disorder, since it is the deliberate killing of an innocent human being.
>
> ...This evaluation of the *morality of abortion* is to be applied also to the recent forms of intervention on human embryos which...inevitably involve the killing of those embryos.
>
> ...*This moral condemnation also regards* procedures that exploit living human embryos..."produced"...by in vitro fertilization...The killing of innocent human creatures, even if carried out to help others, constitutes an absolutely unacceptable act.

Donum Vitae (Sacred Congregation for the Doctrine of the Faith, 1987) also makes a distinction between procured abortion and the destruction of human embryos in an artificial environment outside of a woman's body (emphasis mine):

> In the usual practice of in vitro fertilization, not all of the embryos are transferred to the woman's body; some are destroyed. *Just as the Church condemns induced abortion*, so she also forbids acts against the life of these human beings.

Again, *Donum Vitae* (Sacred Congregation for the Doctrine of the Faith, 1987) distinguishes the destruction of these embryos from procured abortion, even while acknowledging they are linked by being two species of homicide (emphasis mine):

> But even in a situation in which every precaution were taken to avoid the death of human embryos, homologous IVF and ET dissociates from the conjugal act the actions which are directed to human fertilization. For this reason the very nature of homologous IVF and ET also must be taken into account, *even abstracting from the link with procured abortion.*

For consistency with my definition of abortion at the beginning of this section, I believe it important to distinguish abortion proper from the destruction of embryos that exist outside of a woman's body in an artificial environment. Abortion proper is a medical or chemical intervention that intends to destroy an unborn child in a woman's body, whereas the term "sin of abortion" was introduced in *Dignitas Personae* (Sacred Congregation for the Doctrine of the Faith, 2008) and can apply more broadly to any destruction of an embryo or fetus at any point from conception onward. For clarity, I propose to define particular terms that refer to specific categories of the term "abortion" and those that do not.

Categories of Abortion

Abortion (induced, procured, direct, etc.): the direct termination of a pregnancy, from conception to birth, with the intent to destroy a human life; "every act tending directly to destroy human life in the womb" (Pope John Paul II, 1995).

Embryo reduction: in reference to the transfer of multiple embryos into a woman's womb, "a procedure in which embryos or fetuses in the womb are directly exterminated", "an intentional selective abortion" (Sacred Congregation for the Doctrine of the Faith, 2008; see also Lanfranchi, 2024).

Selective abortion: applying specifically to embryos in the womb, "the deliberate and direct elimination of one or more innocent human beings in the initial phase of their existence" (Sacred Congregation for the Doctrine of the Faith, 2008).

Sin of abortion: "the deliberate and direct killing, by whatever means it is carried out, of a human being in the initial phase of his or her existence, extending from conception to birth" (Pope John Paul II, 1995). The penalties in Canon Law apply equally to the destruction of embryos outside of a woman's body in an artificial environment as they do to abortion (Pope John Paul II, 1988; see also Sacred Congregation for the Doctrine of the Faith, 2008).

Loss of an Unborn Child Not to be Considered an Abortion

In vitro extermination (extermination of embryos produced in vitro): the destruction of human embryos outside of a woman's body in an artificial environment (Sacred Congregation for the Doctrine of the Faith, 1987; Pope John Paul II, 1995); has the character of the sin of abortion.

Miscarriage: the spontaneous natural termination of a pregnancy resulting in the loss of an embryo or fetus from the uterus during the first 20 weeks of gestational age, also strangely referred to as a "spontaneous abortion" (Medical News Today, 2018; MedlinePlus, 2025).

Stillbirth: the spontaneous natural termination of a pregnancy resulting in the loss of an embryo or fetus from the uterus after 20 weeks of gestational age and before birth (U.S. Centers for Disease Control and Prevention, 2025)

Unintended pregnancy loss: miscarriage, embryo death (loss), fetal demise, complete hydatidiform mole, certain partial hydatidiform moles, certain ectopic implantations that terminate naturally, others (AAPC, 2025)

The reason for citing the Magisterial teaching and for listing the definitions above is to: (1) emphasize that human life, human dignity, and human rights must be considered to begin at conception; (2) as such, no one has the authority to violate this life, this dignity, and these rights from conception onward; (3) in vitro embryos are considered by the Church to be equally alive with human dignity and human rights as born children; (4) the destruction of an in vitro embryo has a moral character on par with the ending of a human life by induced abortion.

An Ambiguity in *Dignitas Personae*?

Dignitas Personae (Sacred Congregation for the Doctrine of the Faith, 2008) suggests that the intentional destruction of a human embryo outside of a woman's body in an artificial environment be classified as an abortion. This doctrinal instruction refers not only to abortion proper (destruction of human life in the womb), but also extends this term to include my proposed term *in vitro extermination*, which does not refer to the destruction of human life inside a woman's body, but instead specifically refers to the destruction of human embryos outside of a woman's body in an artificial environment. The doctrinal instruction applies the following terms to in vitro extermination: "abortion", "selective abortion", "act of abortion". In Paragraph 21 of this doctrinal instruction, the term "selective abortion" is used in reference to embryos inside of a woman's womb, whereas in Paragraph 22 the same term is applied to embryos outside of a woman's body in an artificial environment. In Paragraphs 16 and 22 the doctrinal instruction applies the term "abortion" to embryos outside of a woman's body in an artificial environment. For consistency with previous Magisterial documents, I would prefer that a distinction be made between the killing of embryos inside of a woman's body and the extermination of embryos outside of a woman's body in an artificial environment. As seen above, previous Magisterial documents did indeed make a distinction between abortion proper and the destruction of embryos outside of a woman's body in an artificial environment. I assume that the distinction was made in these documents to avoid confusion regarding longstanding understandings of pregnancy and abortion. These Magisterial documents *link* to the immorality of abortion the immorality of the killing of embryos produced by in vitro fertilization and existing outside of a woman's body in an artificial environment, but they do not classify this type of homicide as abortion. Both types of homicide constitute different species of murder. Within the scope of my proposed definitions above, I consider it a misnomer to refer to the destruction of a human embryo existing outside of a woman's body in an artificial environment as an abortion.

Embryo Adoption

Many human embryos conceived in a laboratory environment are preserved in the frozen state. For example, during a 10-year period from 2004 through 2013, 1,945,548 such embryos were preserved this way (Christianson, 2020). Is an embryo conceived in a laboratory a human person? The nature of a human person is discussed in some detail in Chapter 9. Here is how the Catholic Church answers this question in *Dignitas Personae* (Sacred Congregation for the Doctrine of the Faith, 2008):

> Although the presence of the spiritual soul cannot be observed experimentally, the conclusions of science regarding the human embryo give "a valuable indication for discerning by the use of reason a personal presence at the moment of the first appearance of a human life: how could a human individual not be a human person?".

If these frozen embryos are truly human persons, as the Catholic Church believes, then they have human dignity and because of this, they have the right to live. If they have the same right to live as born children have, then they deserve to be treated with the same respect as born children. Is there anything standing in the way of a man and woman in a state of matrimony adopting these innocent embryonic children, regardless of how they were conceived?

Effectiveness of In Vitro Fertilization Versus Natural Family Planning

In Endnote 2 of a 2025 open letter to Vice President J.D. Vance, Sister Renee Mirkes offered a few statistics about the effectiveness of methods of *Natural Family Planning* versus IVF (Mirkes, 2025). Natural Family Planning makes use of the natural fertility cycle in the woman and applies proven methods of science to either enhance the likelihood of achieving pregnancy or lessen this likelihood. For nearly four decades, the Saint Paul VI Institute for the Study of Human Reproduction has been treating infertility as a medical condition that in many cases can be treated with procedures developed at the Institute. When the Institute's methods of

Natural Family Planning are used to enhance the likelihood of achieving pregnancy, the results are encouraging. For example, the Institute reported in 2004 that in a study of the cumulative pregnancy rate for 1,054 infertile women who utilized the Institute's "NaPro" infertility protocols, over 60% of these patients achieved pregnancy within 24 months, and nearly 70% within 36 months. The Endnote compares these statistics to a much lower pregnancy rate from IVF.

To the extent that human persons are in reality the result of creative acts of God and are sustained in existence and relationship by the care of God for His creation, artificial human procreation and contraception are to be avoided. It may happen that an unmarried woman is faced with an unplanned pregnancy. If she finds herself unable to properly care for the child, then foster care or adoption are options. Adoption or foster parenting are also options for those couples who are joined together in sacred matrimony but incapable of natural generation of children by morally-sound means.

What about those married couples who for serious reasons find that they must space the births of children, but who believe that extended periods of abstinence from conjugal relations would harm their marital relationship? Natural Family Planning can help these couples, too. When used to regulate the spacings of births, Natural Family Planning aligns with the teachings of St. Paul and the dual purposes of the conjugal embrace. From 1 Corinthians 7:5 (NAB):

> Do not deprive each other, except perhaps by mutual consent for a time, to be free for prayer, but then return to one another, so that Satan may not tempt you through your lack of self-control.

Natural Family Planning meets the criteria of the dual purposes of the conjugal embrace by being properly unitive and by being open to the possibility of pregnancy. Although Natural Family Planning can be an effective method for the prudent spacing of births, it is not 100% effective at doing so. Because pregnancy remains possible when the method is used, the couple's openness to procreation leaves room for God to act if He so chooses to allow a child to be conceived during any given conjugal embrace.

CHAPTER 8

A BRIEF NOTE ON THE NATURE OF THE ONE TRUE GOD AND HIS RELATIONSHIP TO MAN

What follows is an attempt to give a brief insight into the greatest mystery of Christianity: the *ontological* nature of God. According to Catholic understanding, God's nature is only partially comprehensible to the human mind. Human explanations of God's nature do not contradict reason but are unable to provide the fullness of what can be known about God both in human temporal existence and on the spiritual plane. God exists in a realm called heaven, a glorious kingdom that we know something about, but not all that much. The portal to heaven for almost all people who have ever lived is death. I, nor any human person, can fully visualize the life the Christian believes will appertain after death for one who strives to live in accordance with revelation and right reason and to believe what is known about God through special revelation and nature since the beginning of human history until now.

Why does this matter? Because if there is in reality the type of afterlife believed by Christians to exist, then the rational and prudent person would choose to live his temporal life in a such a way as to become part of this vision of the afterlife after dying. Pascal's wager addresses this question and draws a conclusion that I believe is unassailable by any thinking person who knows the difference between good and evil, right and wrong. Everyone wants comfort, security, and true peace in this life. The Christian believes these needs can be met in a most perfect way in the afterlife. Not only that, but we reason that if God is just, as divine revelation intends to demonstrate, then injustice suffered by a person in this life, when borne with the patience and perseverance that Christ exemplified in His life on earth, will be compensated with reward in the next life.

According to my Catholic understanding, heaven is not an earthly place, but a "dwelling place of the blessed", outside of the physical universe and beyond its limits (Hontheim, 1910). The inhabitants of this place are in the presence of God. The Catholic faith teaches that at least two of these inhabitants left earthly life with their bodies: Jesus Christ and His mother, Mary. While on earth, their bodies were physical and subject to the afflictions that we from time to time suffer. However, on leaving this physical existence, their bodies were transfigured into a condition or state known as *glorified*. This glorified state is considered in some sense material, but whether it consists of atoms and molecules is not known. I think it unlikely that this would be the case, in as much as heaven is eternal, i.e., not subject to the passage of time and to the types of change that happen as time progresses. Perhaps the best way to think of heaven is not in three-dimensional spatial coordinates or even in time, but in reference to "where" God is—outside of space as we know it and of time. That being said, it is also believed that God is often unexpectedly close to us here and now in a spiritual sense. According to my understanding of divine revelation, God can and will at some point in the future, as we reckon it, create a new home for the people in heaven that will manifest perfect peace, complete security, and the comfort of knowing who God is face to face. The condition of knowing God face to face, in Himself as He exists, is referred to by Catholic theology as the *beatific vision.* This vision is considered a condition of perfect joy, belonging, and peace.

Assuming that the reader of this treatise would aspire to embrace this concept of afterlife, it then makes sense to explain what kind of God would exist and make this possible. Unfortunately, as noted in the beginning of this chapter, the human mind can only partially comprehend the fullness of God's reality and existence. The best it can do is to reason from what is seen, heard, felt, smelled, and tasted in its temporal existence, and from what can be known by divine revelation from God. We reason that God exists as a being with definable attributes, such as omnipotence, omniscience, immutability, ultimate goodness, ultimate perfection, ultimate charity, and other attributes that are described in standard sources on the Christian faith and even in ancient Greek philosophy. Other religions stemming from the true religion of Adam and Eve, Noah, and other early patriarchs of biblical record retain and maintain knowledge of these attributes and can serve as distant lights which can lead to the fullness of truth.

Christians refer to the "fullness of truth" as a divine and human person—Jesus Christ. Jesus Christ (or "Jesus the Christ") made His appearance to men as God on earth and found His human origin in the second greatest mystery in Christianity: the *Incarnation.* To explain the mystery of the Incarnation is to delve into the mystery of the Godhead. Found in divine revelation is convincing evidence that God exists as three divine Persons (but ***not*** as three gods), distinguishable from one another by their relationship to one another. The Athanasian Creed, Nicene Creed, and other early sources of belief in the nature of the Godhead explain in some detail what is known about God and the relationship between the three Persons of God, as well as brief references to His relationship with people in the temporal sphere.

> In the beginning was the Word [*Logos*], and the Word was with God, and the Word was God. [John 1:1, NAB]

St. John in his Gospel goes on to describe the Logos as the creator of reality external to Himself, the source of eternal life, the light of men, and the One who is capable of empowering men to become adopted children of God. The term "children of God" needs elaboration because it reveals much about the relationship of God to man. I quote here from St. Paul's letter to the Romans (8:14-25, NAB):

> For those who are led by the Spirit of God are children of God. For you did not receive a spirit of slavery to fall back into fear, but you received a spirit of adoption, through which we cry, "Abba, Father!" The Spirit itself bears witness with our spirit that we are children of God, and if children, then heirs, heirs of God and joint heirs with Christ, if only we suffer with him so that we may also be glorified with him. I consider that the sufferings of this present time are as nothing compared with the glory to be revealed for us. For creation awaits with eager expectation the revelation of

> the children of God; for creation was made subject to futility, not of its own accord but because of the one who subjected it, in hope that creation itself would be set free from slavery to corruption and share in the glorious freedom of the children of God. We know that all creation is groaning in labor pains even until now; and not only that, but we ourselves, who have the firstfruits of the Spirit, we also groan within ourselves as we wait for adoption, the redemption of our bodies. For in hope we were saved. Now hope that sees for itself is not hope. For who hopes for what one sees? But if we hope for what we do not see, we wait with endurance.

Much can be learned about the place of man in God's creation from this excerpt. There is a *Spirit of God* who leads men to the Father. The children of God live in a *spirit of adoption* and are heirs to an eternal inheritance of freedom from suffering and loss. The children of God are not left with nothing but hope; rather they are joined through sanctifying grace in this life to Jesus Christ who is the refulgence of the glory of God the Father, "the very imprint of His being" (Hebrews 1:3, NAB). Heaven is the ultimate freedom from slavery to whatever binds people to sin in this life and from whatever physical ailments afflict people in this life. The "firstfruits of the Spirit" is another way of expressing *justification* ("spirit of adoption") before God in time (on earth). Justification is the spiritual and moral state before God that allows a man at death to be destined for heaven. It represents the transformation "of the sinner from the state of unrighteousness to the state of holiness and sonship of God" (Pohle, 1910). We presently hope as children of God for eternal adoption to live in a future eternal world where redeemed souls join back with their own bodies at the *general resurrection.* At the general resurrection, the bodies of the justified will be transformed in a material sense to be capable of living in an eternal world. The eternal adoption as children of God is called *eternal salvation. Endurance* (patience through time) is a critical quality for remaining in a state of justification and eventually attaining eternal salvation in the next life. Endurance leads to *final perseverance,* .which is to remain in a state of sanctifying grace until the end of life (Sollier, 1911).

I was reminded that a new "place" will be created by God for those to live in who have attained eternal salvation after the general resurrection (D. Bouchard, personal communication, .15 August 2025). Here are some Scriptural references to this new creation:

> For there shall be a new heaven and a new earth. [Isaiah 65:17, Brenton Septuagint translation]

> For we know that, when our earthly house of this habitation is dissolved, we have a building of God, a house not made with hands, eternal in heaven. [2 Corinthians 5:17, Catholic Public Domain Version]

> But according to his promise we await new heavens and a new earth in which righteousness dwells. [2 Peter 3:13, NAB]

> I saw the new heaven and the new earth. For the first heaven and the first earth passed away. [Revelation 21:1, Catholic Public Domain Version]

The Christian conception of God is radically different from the Jewish, Muslim, Hindu, pantheistic, and other conceptions. According to Christian theology, the Godhead manifests to men in eternal existence as ***one*** God in a *Trinity* of divine Persons: God the Father, God the Son (the eternal Logos), and God the Holy Spirit. Evidence for this is alluded to in the excerpt above from St. Paul's letter to the Romans. The Catholic Encyclopedia includes an extensive discussion on the Trinity and cites St. Matthew's Gospel as the definitive Scriptural evidence of the Trinitarian nature of God (Joyce, 1912):

> Go, therefore, and make disciples of all nations, baptizing them in the name of the Father, and of the Son, and of the holy Spirit. [Matthew 28:19, NAB]

But this verse is not the only evidence. An inference to the Trinity can be found in Genesis 1:1-2 (English Standard Version), which says the following:

> In the beginning, God created the heavens and the earth. The earth was without form and void, and darkness was over the face of the deep. And the Spirit of God was hovering over the face of the waters.

St. Augustine has much to say about "the beginning", and since I usually find his first interpretations of biblical verses intriguing, I will dwell for a moment on his first interpretation of this phrase (Augustine of Hippo, 415). This interpretation builds upon the first verse in the Gospel of St. John, quoted above: "In the beginning was the Word, and the Word was with God, and the Word was God". St. Augustine suggests a strong correlation between "the beginning" and "the Word" that was God. If we write "the beginning" = "the Word", it can been seen that "the beginning" could be considered another name for "the Word" that was God. In as much as "the Word" in Christianity is the primary name of the second divine Person of the Trinity, "the beginning" could be used to place "the Word" in the opening verses (Genesis 1:1-2) of the Bible:

> In the Word, God created the heavens and the earth. The earth was without form and void, and darkness was over the face of the deep. And the Spirit of God was hovering over the face of the waters.

On consideration of the second verse ("...the Spirit of God was hovering over the face of the waters "), St. Augustine in his first interpretation of "the Spirit of God" considers this Spirit to be the Holy Spirit of the Trinity. In as much as God the Father is known as the First divine Person of the Trinity (most often referred to simply as "God") and God the Son the Second, God the Holy Spirit is the Third. When a Christian refers in prayer to God, it is generally to God the Father that he prays, unless he specifically cites another Person of the Trinity. Thus St. Augustine sees evidence of the Trinity in the opening verses of Genesis.

The three divine Persons of the Godhead have been from all eternity purely spiritual in substance. God the Son is said to find His origin in eternity by *generation from the Father*. The name "Logos" ("Word") is descriptive of the visible actions wrought by the Second Person of the Trinity, and He is the Person who entered the temporal sphere and *assumed* a human nature in the event mentioned above—the Incarnation. In Christianity, the Incarnation is the miracle whereby the Holy Spirit "overshadowed" a young woman (Mary, the mother of Jesus Christ) and in an unknown way facilitated the joining of the Word with a human embryo. At the moment of conception, the Word formed a physical bond between the Godhead and humanity. After nine months He was born as a man. God is said to have become one of us, and His name is Jesus Christ. Jesus Christ is both man and the Second Person of the Trinity, God. In technical language, the Second Person of the Trinity assumed a human nature in the person of Jesus Christ in what is called the *hypostatic union*.

> And the Word became flesh, and he lived among us, and we saw his glory, glory like that of an only-begotten son from the Father, full of grace and truth. [John 1:14, Catholic Public Domain Version]

In case you may be asking if there is evidence in the Bible that Jesus Christ knew He was God and claimed to be God, St. Mark's Gospel provides this evidence:

> Again the high priest asked him, and said to him: Art thou the Christ the Son of the blessed God? And Jesus said to him: I am. [Mark 14:61-62, Rheims New Testament]

The original Greek words for "I am" are Ἐγώ εἰμι, which is the name that God answered to in the Old Testament:

> God replied to Moses: I am who I am. Then he added: This is what you will tell the Israelites: I AM has sent me to you. [Exodus 3:14, NAB]

A Jewish translation of the Old Testament from Hebrew into Greek occurred in the third century B.C. and is known as the Septuagint, or LXX. As found in the LXX, the Greek words for "I am" in Exodus 3:14 are Ἐγώ εἰμι, exactly the same words as are found in St. Mark's Gospel. It is clear from Mark 14:63-64 that the high priest knew that Jesus was claiming to be God, because on hearing Jesus utter "I am", the high priest tore his garments and declared that Jesus had committed the capital infraction of blasphemy:

> At that the high priest tore his garments and said, "What further need have we of witnesses? You have heard the blasphemy." [NAB]

Corroborating evidence that Jesus knew He was God and claimed to be God is found in the Gospel of St. John:

> Jesus said to them, "Amen, amen, I say to you, before Abraham came to be, I AM." So they picked up stones to throw at him. [John 8:58-59, NAB]

In St. John's account, Jesus not only calls himself by God's name, but He calls himself the God of Abraham. The God of Abraham is unequivocally the God who Jesus' Jewish audience worshipped. At Jesus equating Himself to the God of Abraham, His audience rose up and attempted to stone Him for the sin of blasphemy.

I will now try to explain by heuristic means one way in which the finite human intellect can partially grasp the nature of one God in three divine Persons. This explanation is useful only insofar as analogy can shed some small light upon the unexplainable. Consider the power of a word uttered by a man. For example, the word "Charge!" can be used to start the battle in a war. The word "peace" can be used to end a war. The word "racist" can end a person's career. The word "ultraconservative" can be used in "scholarly" publications to denigrate a point of view that the authors disagree with. In each of these cases, words influence or even end lives—words can have power. Consider as well that a word uttered by me is mine—I own it. Even if billions of other people utter that same word, when it is uttered by me it is mine. Now consider the all-powerful God the Father uttering a Word in eternity. We can imagine that if our own word can invoke a powerful response, God's Word can do infinitely more. This is a way in which the Second Person of the Trinity may be understood as being of the Father, one with the Father by personal possession, representative of the

Father, and an "express image" (from Hebrews 1:3 in alternate translation from the Greek) of the Father (Green, 1988).

But how is the connection expressly made between the Second Person of the Trinity and Jesus Christ? I find St. Augustine's first interpretation again intriguing. Even though there is argument about the exact meaning of the beginning words (Tὴν ἀρχὴν) of Jesus' answer in the following verse (John 8:25, Rheims New Testament), the interpretation of St. Augustine is as insightful as it is imaginative.

> They said therefore to him: Who art thou? Jesus said to them: The beginning, who also speak unto you.

In this verse from the Rheims New Testament one might see the self-identification of Jesus with "the beginning", in other words, His self-identification with the Word.

The Bible is seen in this interpretation to provide evidence in support of the Christian mystery of the Sacred Trinity. The standard description of the Ontological Trinity is the following: the Father loves the Son, the Son loves the Father, and the bond of love is so strong that a third Person, the Holy Spirit, exists to communicate these two relationships. This is the essence of the one God's internal relationships among the Persons of the Trinity. It might be said that God the Father utters a Word that He is bound to in a holy spirit (i.e., in a manner that manifests the 3rd Person of the Trinity). Among the best illuminations of the Trinity is the Athanasian Creed, reproduced in partial excerpt from the Catholic Encyclopedia in the Appendix.

God's relationship to man, on the other hand, is known as the *Economic Trinity*. The Catechism of the Catholic Church (n. 236) says that the Economic Trinity consists of: "all the works by which God reveals himself and communicates his life" to man. God interacts with man in a variety of unseen ways—examples include through faith, grace, prayer, miracles, and other signs. According to Catholic theology, *baptism* effects the state of justification in the one who receives this sacrament. With justification comes the infusion of the supernatural virtues of faith in God, hope in God's eternal adoption as children of God, and charity, or love of man for his Creator. Justification can take place at any point in time after birth. The virtue of faith can embrace understanding when a person attains the age of reason (commonly assumed to be 7 years of age in persons with normal intellects). Faith is an interesting communion between God and man, and it is able to expand once a person is able to reason about the natural and supernatural worlds. How would an unbaptized person who is capable of reasoning become justified and acquire the virtue of faith? Justification takes place in unbaptized persons who have attained both the age of reason and the use of reason through a process detailed in the sixth session of the Council of Trent on 13 January 1547 (Schroeder, 1978):

> It is furthermore declared that in adults the beginning of that justification must proceed from the predisposing grace of God through Jesus Christ, that is, from His vocation, whereby, without any merits on their part, they are called; that they who by sin had been cut off from God, may be disposed through His quickening and helping

> grace to convert themselves to their own justification by freely assenting to and cooperating with that grace; so that, while God touches the heart of man through the illumination of the Holy Ghost, man himself neither does absolutely nothing while receiving that inspiration, since he can also reject it, nor yet is he able by his own free will and without the grace of God to move himself to justice in His sight.

Thus it is seen that faith comes by grace to those who allow God to move themselves with His grace to righteousness. As mentioned in Chapter 4, grace is a free and undeserved assistance from God "to respond to his call to become children of God" (Catechism of the Catholic Church, n. 1996). Catholics identify two species of grace: sanctifying (habitual) and actual. *Sanctifying grace* is a participation in the life of God, a mysterious share in the Ontological Trinity. *Actual graces* are gifts received through God's intervention that assist in the work of sanctification (Catechism of the Catholic Church, nn. 1999-2000).

CHAPTER 9

ON DOUBT AND UNCERTAINTY IN THE MATTERS OF HUMAN CONCEPTION AND PREGNANCY

Doubt and Uncertainty in General, with Examples

What is *doubt*? Wiktionary says this about doubt: "To be undecided about; to lack confidence in". A more precise definition may be found in the Catholic Encyclopedia (Sharpe, 1909):

> A state in which the mind is suspended between two contradictory propositions and unable to assent to either of them. Any number of alternative propositions on the same subject may be in doubt at the same time; but, strictly speaking, the doubt is attached separately to each one, as between the proposition and its contradictory, i.e. each proposition may or may not be true. Doubt is opposed to certitude, or the adhesion of the mind to a proposition without misgiving as to its truth; and again to opinion, or a mental adhesion to a proposition together with such a misgiving. ...It should be observed that doubt is a purely subjective condition; i.e., it belongs only to the mind which has to judge of facts, and has no application to the facts themselves. A proposition or theory which is commonly called doubtful is, therefore, one as to which sufficient evidence to

> determine assent is not forthcoming; in itself it must be either true or false. Theories which have at one time been regarded as doubtful for want of sufficient evidence, frequently become certainly true or false by reason of the discovery of fresh evidence.

Wiktionary defines *uncertainty* as: "Doubt; the condition of being uncertain or without conviction." Wikipedia (20 June 2023) expanded on this definition:

> Uncertainty refers to epistemic situations involving imperfect or unknown information. It applies to predictions of future events, to physical measurements that are already made, or to the unknown.

In simpler terms, Wikipedia defines uncertainty this way:

> The lack of certainty, a state of limited knowledge where it is impossible to exactly describe the existing state, a future outcome, or more than one possible outcome.

Why a discussion about doubt? Because there are few prudential decisions, measurements, observations, or conclusions that can be entirely and absolutely free from doubt or uncertainty. Examples of this abound. Measurement with a ruler is only precise to the nearest half gradation. This is known as the uncertainty of a linear measurement. Weather forecasts always carry a certain degree of uncertainty. A forecast can suggest rain tomorrow, but by morning the next day the forecast can change to clear skies all day. Every year we see uncertainty in climate variability. Will September be warmer or cooler this year than August? Will August be warmer or cooler this year than last year? Will August be warmer or cooler than it was 100 years ago? Will this year be warmer or cooler than it was 5,000 years ago? Even in the realm of moral decisions, doubt and uncertainty are present in a prudential sense. This chapter is not a philosophical look into doubt and uncertainty, nor even a theological one. It is an attempt to apply common sense to situations where doubt cannot be overcome.

My first example of doubt is faced by many who commute by automobile to and from work in a large city. In my own case, during the majority of years that I worked downtown, but lived outside of the city, I needed to commute approximately 15 miles by the shortest route each way. I was fortunate there were three interstate highways through the city, which allowed a greater variety of travel efficiencies and routes. Even city streets were an option when traffic was heavy due to an accident or other event on the highways. My decision about which route to take home was always made in the light of doubt and uncertainty as defined above. Each of my decisions about which route to take was *prudential*, not *moral.* Why? Because in most cases the route I chose had no bearing on the divine law or the natural law. My choice was a choice of convenience, greatest safety and efficiency, and automobile and environmental considerations. If I chose well, I could be home from work in as little as 20 minutes. If I chose poorly, the trip could take up to a couple of hours. There was no moral "right" or "wrong" in almost every decision that I could make about which route to take.

There were only better outcomes and worse outcomes. I define moral "right" or "wrong" as alignment or nonalignment with God's standards as communicated to man through the Catholic Church and the natural law. The natural law can be thought of as the rule of conduct prescribed to us by our Creator in the nature He has endowed us and "manifested to us by the purely natural medium of reason" (Fox, 1910).

The choice of which Mass to attend is my second example of doubt, an example which is a bit more subjective than my first example, but which in some cases requires a moral, not prudential, decision. In my limited experience of attending Mass at fewer than one hundred different parishes in the United States and abroad, I have found personally (subjectively) satisfying and unsatisfying styles of conduct by those serving at Mass or by those in attendance in the pews. In the unsatisfying cases, I have at times needed to exercise a form of Catholic detachment because of various types of mistake or distraction, such as a failure to adhere to the rubrics, a lack of fidelity to the required readings, the choice and volume of music, the noise level before and after Mass, the noise level and other distractions during Mass, the style and message of homilies, or because of other considerations. Russell Shaw defines Catholic detachment as follows (Shaw, 2016):

> To be detached, to practice detachment, is to establish and maintain a relation to everything and everybody in one's life according to which all things are valued by how much they help or hinder us in our relationship with God, the imitation of Christ, and the service of other people.

In extreme cases of liturgical mistakes or various combinations of distractions during Mass, a moral decision may be necessary. At first, this decision is prudential because of doubt about my own perception of the liturgical irregularities and the frequency and severity of distractions. However, after repeated exposure and confirmation of either laxity or the intent to offer a Mass which is abusive to liturgical standards, a moral decision must be made. The basis for this moral decision is contingent upon the outcome of consultations with the liturgical leadership. If these consultations do not result in correction of the liturgical abuse or of the failure to discipline, then two courses of action may be considered: find a non-abusive parish, or if this is not possible, exercise Catholic detachment in order to maintain a proper relationship with God and to better imitate Christ.

A Diseased Uterus

The next example is a situation of doubt based on a purely moral decision. Imagine a medical problem in which a woman was just diagnosed with a malignant cancer of the uterus that has a high likelihood of killing her *within the next 2 months.* The moral decision the physician and woman would have to make is whether or not to remove the cancerous uterus. If the uterus is removed, an organ is lost, and normal childbearing becomes impossible. If the uterus stays, the woman dies. Pretty easy decision, right? "Do no harm" comes to mind, which in this case means "do lesser harm". In this case of proportionate evils, leaving the uterus in place certainly does the greater harm to the life of the woman. Now consider a twist on this scenario. The woman found out she is in the beginning stage of pregnancy (e.g., *a few days into the pregnancy*) the day before receiving the bad news about the cancer. Should the same medical procedure of removing the cancerous uterus take place? What are the moral implications?

Catholic moral teaching makes it clear that abortion is a grave moral evil under *every* circumstance. Should the woman with the cancerous uterus consent to an abortion? This is the wrong question, since procured abortion is gravely immoral in all situations. The proper question to ask is: "Should the woman undergo the same medical procedure that would have been performed had she not been pregnant?" Consider the facts as they exist today: (1) an unborn child of fewer than 20 weeks gestation cannot survive outside its mother's womb, (2) the woman will die without the medical procedure, (3) the death of two persons is a greater physical evil than the death of one person, (4) the fate of the unborn child's soul is known only to a good God who delivers positive punishment upon no one who is free of personal sin (cf. Aquinas, 1274; Toner, 1910). Add to these considerations the fact that the medical procedure will not succeed *because* of the death of the child, but *because* of the removal of the uterus. The death of the child is an unintended consequence of a procedure that would have been performed if the woman were not pregnant. In this situation (days into the pregnancy), the woman and her physician are morally free to choose to go through with the medical procedure because the principle of double effect applies. If she did not agree, both she and the unborn child would die before the pregnancy had progressed to three months from conception.

The Eternal Word Television Network (EWTN) has an article in its online library that addresses this same situation and is titled "Indirect Abortion" (Healy, 2025). I find this title unfortunate because of the use of the word "abortion". Terms such as these are one of the reasons for the writing of this treatise—to redefine terminology in order to lessen possible confusion about the nature of certain medical procedures that can impact unborn life in the womb. Although the article is very informative and applies the principle of double effect in a manner similar to the example above, I think a change in terminology is needed. I might suggest a term like "therapeutic excision" to refer to the surgical operation and "uterine" to refer to the affected organ: "uterine therapeutic excision". Because the woman is pregnant, even more specificity would be helpful, even if it does extend the name of the procedure even longer: "uterine therapeutic excision with child".

Catholicism considers it important to baptize an unborn child who is removed from the womb prematurely and dies because he is too young to be saved by current technology. Baptism of such a child would guarantee justification and a destination for heaven on dying. If baptism cannot be administered due to ignorance, neglect, indifference. or other cause, the eternal fate of the unborn child is not so easy to discern. The Catechism of the Catholic Church (n. 1257) emphasizes the necessity of baptism this way:

> The Church does not know of any means other than Baptism that assures entry into eternal beatitude; this is why she takes care not to neglect the mission she has received

from the Lord to see that all who can be baptized are "reborn of water and the Spirit."

Speculation about the state of existence of the soul of an unborn child who dies without baptism has been going on for centuries. Up until the middle of the 20th century, Catholic catechesis taught that eternal natural happiness is guaranteed for such children (Aquinas, 1274; Toner, 1910), but more recent theology suggests there may be reason to hope for the possibility of supernatural happiness (International Theological Commission, 2007). The Catechism of the Catholic Church suggests this possibility:

> God has bound salvation to the sacrament of baptism, but he himself is not bound by his sacraments. [n. 1257]

> As regards children who have died without baptism, the Church can only entrust them to the mercy of God. [n. 1261]

Healy (2025) provides guidance on how Catholic medical personnel (and anyone else who chooses to do what the Church does for the soul of the tiny patient) should react to the unborn child as soon as the diseased uterus is removed from the mother's body. He says that a basin of water should be set nearby beforehand so that the child may be baptized as soon as his skin is accessible by water. The child should be removed from the uterus and from any sac or membrane that may be present, and then immediately baptized either by pouring the water on the skin or by immersion if the child is very small. The proper form should be used while the water is in contact with the skin: St. Matthew's Gospel, verse 28:19 (see Chapter 8).

Ectopic Pregnancy

Now to a situation which can pose a greater moral difficulty for those who value human life as much as God does. It is a form of pregnancy and a medical condition with a descriptive name: ectopic pregnancy. This medical condition (Kirk, 2014) is defined as a *complication of pregnancy* in which the embryo implants outside the *normal uterine cavity*, or corpus of the uterus (Cleveland Clinic, 2024a, 2024b; Sivalingam, 2011)—an out of place ("ectopic") implantation. As a complication of pregnancy, this condition represents a medical problem that should be followed by a physician throughout the pregnancy (Cleveland Clinic, 2023; Office on Women's Health, 2025; John Hopkins Medicine, 2025; Stickler, 2016; University of Rochester, 2025). In a review published in 2014 of 32 studies of conservative treatments for ectopic pregnancies, the review article's authors note in the abstract that an ectopic pregnancy can become risky and is the leading cause of maternal death in the first trimester of pregnancy (Cecchino, 2014). On the basis of reviews such as this one, it is seen that this complication of pregnancy can be a serious medical condition that should be treated in a timely manner. But not only can it be a serious medical condition that would need to be treated in a timely manner, its rate of incidence has been found to be increasing (Raine-Bennett, 2022;

Francis, 2024). In fact, Vadakekut (2025) reported that in vitro fertilization increases the likelihood of ectopic implantation.

As seen in Chapter 7 and in the example of the cancerous uterus above, a specific goal of this treatise is to propose and to speak as an *advocate* for greater precision in definitions and medical terminology related to: (1) pregnancy and its ending, (2) complications of pregnancy, and (3) embryos in artificial environments outside of a woman's body. Precision in terminology can be capable of tipping the balance towards life in discussions of doubt and uncertainty in the matters of pregnancy, medical conditions, and the responses to them. Even though I am a nonspecialist in medicine, philosophy, and bioethics, I do have experience in precise observations and terminology.

In order to distinguish ectopic complications of pregnancy from a normal healthy pregnancy, it is important to consider a current, commonly-used definition of pregnancy and compare it to my proposed definition in Chapter 7. Here is the way the U.S. National Institutes of Health (NIH) website defines pregnancy (About Pregnancy, 2024):

> Pregnancy is the term used to describe the period in which a fetus develops inside a woman's womb or uterus. ...The events that lead to pregnancy begin with conception, in which a sperm penetrates an egg. The fertilized egg (called a zygote) then travels through the woman's Fallopian tube to the uterus, where it implants itself in the uterine wall. The zygote is made up of a cluster of cells that later form the fetus.

The definition that I proposed in Chapter 7 is:

> Pregnancy is the term used to describe the condition of carrying developing offspring within a woman's body.

This definition expands the location of pregnancy beyond the uterine cavity to include implantations of an early-stage embryo in other locations in the woman's body. As noted in Chapter 7, four medical dictionaries agree with this definition (Gacek, 2009), even though they use somewhat different ways to express the same concept; e.g.:

> the condition of having a developing embryo or fetus in the body, after union of an ovum and spermatozoon

> the gestational process, comprising the growth and development within a woman of a new individual from conception through the embryonic and fetal periods to birth

> the state of a female after conception until the birth of the child

> the condition of having a developing embryo or fetus in the body, after successful conception

The difference between the NIH and other popular definitions of pregnancy versus mine and those found in the cited medical dictionaries is that in my proposed definition and in those cited in the medical dictionaries, pregnancy begins at conception within a woman's body, whereas in the NIH definition pregnancy begins at implantation in the uterus. This difference bears greatly on arguments for and against contraception and abortion.

It was recently pointed out to me that some believe that the term "pregnancy" should be extended to apply to embryos that are created and kept outside of a woman's body in an artificial environment. This seems to extrapolate the concept of "ectopic" a bit too far. Whereas the Catholic Church teaches that human life begins at fertilization, this institution has not taught that pregnancy can exist outside of a woman's body. Here are some examples that demonstrate this. From *Dignitas Personae* (Sacred Congregation for the Doctrine of the Faith, 2008):

> One of the methods for improving the chances of success in techniques of in vitro fertilization is the multiplication of attempts…In this way, should the initial attempt at achieving pregnancy not succeed, the procedure can be repeated or additional pregnancies attempted at a later date.
>
> Some techniques used in artificial procreation, above all the transfer of multiple embryos into the mother's womb, have caused a significant increase in the frequency of multiple pregnancy.
>
> Alongside methods of preventing pregnancy which are, properly speaking, contraceptive, that is, which prevent

conception following from a sexual act, there are other technical means which act after fertilization.

Here is an example from an earlier source (Sacred Congregation for the Doctrine of the Faith, 1987):

> By "surrogate mother", the Instruction means: (a) the woman who carries in pregnancy an embryo implanted in her uterus and who is genetically a stranger to the embryo because it has been obtained through the union of the gametes of "donors". She carries the pregnancy with a pledge to surrender the baby once it is born to the party who commissioned or made the agreement for the pregnancy.

Implantation in a Fallopian Tube

Let us now consider a specific complication of pregnancy where an early-stage embryo implants in a Fallopian tube—an ectopic implantation. This implantation falls within the definition of pregnancy repeated above from Chapter 7. It is often referred to as a "tubal pregnancy" (Papageorgiou, 2025). If this condition were to be diagnosed as certainly fatal in a woman several weeks beyond her last menstrual period, then in order to prevent her death, the condition would need to be remedied when the fetus is too young to survive outside the womb. Would a medical procedure to remove either the embryo from the Fallopian tube or the tube itself constitute an abortion? There are many ways to bring a pregnancy to an end besides abortion. Among these are normal birth, legitimate medical procedures to guard the health of the mother, and complications of pregnancy. Unfortunately, the medical procedure used to remove the tube with the embryo inside is referred to by many as an abortion. Healy (2025) in his article titled "Indirect Abortion" uses the term as well. However, I am more specific in the definition of abortion that I proposed in Chapter 7: the direct termination of a pregnancy, from conception to birth, with the intent to destroy a human life.

Clearly, a tubal pregnancy is not a normal pregnancy, but instead a complication of pregnancy that requires medical attention. It differs from the scenario of a cancerous uterus described above in that even though both are complications of pregnancy, one is a complication due to a preexisting medical condition (Cleveland Clinic, 2022b), while the other is a complication due to the nature of the pregnancy itself. However, the two scenarios are similar in the sense that, like the cancerous uterus that the unborn child is growing within, a child is likewise growing within a Fallopian tube. However, unlike a normal implantation in the uterus, an embryo implanted in a Fallopian tube can begin to cause damage to the tube after implantation. Healy (2025) goes into considerable detail about the early onset and nature of the damage to the Fallopian tube caused by the presence of the embryo implanted in the wrong place. The remedy preferred in this treatise and by medical specialists (Papageorgiou, 2025) for the type of tubal pregnancy that could prove fatal to the woman is to remove the damaged tube or section of the tube *with the embryo inside, not the embryo itself,* but rather the organ that the embryo finds itself inside of. The medical procedure is not an abortion because the intent is to remove the afflicted organ in order to save the life of the mother, not to directly kill the unborn child. As in the case of the diseased uterus, this medical procedure might be called a "tubal therapeutic excision with child". As with the case of the cancerous uterus, the certain death of the unborn child is an unintended consequence of the medical procedure to save the life of the mother. The fate of the embryo would be in God's hands.

If, on the other hand, the embryo itself were attacked directly by surgery or chemical means, then this procedure would be an abortion because the intent would be to directly kill the unborn child. In this situation, the woman's health would be rescued if it were at risk because the child would be removed, but this rescue would come about *by way of the killing of the child.*

I find it unfortunate that some well-meaning Catholics have accepted the strange name of "indirect abortion" for the medical procedure discussed above that removes the tube but does not directly attack the unborn child. It seems to me that this adds a level of unnecessary confusion to the medical procedure. An example of the type of confusion that could be caused by those who label this sort of procedure an abortion is described near the end of Chapter 10.

Other ectopic complications of pregnancy are rarer than a tubal pregnancy. Vadakekut (2025) reported that fewer than 5% of all ectopic pregnancies in the United States are found to occur in the cervix, ovary, uterine cornua, caesarean scar, abdomen, or other locations. Healy (2025) provides guidance in these cases. The first three locations are inside the woman's reproductive system. In situations where the life of the woman is threatened by growth of the unborn child in one of these locations, removal of the damaged organ, as in the case of the tubal pregnancy, can be morally licit according to the conditions of double effect. Implantation and growth of an embryo outside the woman's reproductive system, such as in the abdomen, is a complication beyond the scope of this discussion.

It was suggested to me that an ectopic pregnancy could be surgically transferred from its out-of-place location into the uterus, where it would have a better chance of being born alive. Ben David (2025) in a review article for such a procedure found that although several cases describe success in such transfers, the authors of the review consider the case reports unreliable and the reported results not reproducible. One of these case reports was published by C. J. Wallace in Volume 24 of *Surgery, Gynecology, and Obstetrics*, dated 5 May 1917. This article was reprinted in *The Linacre Quarterly* (Wallace, 1995) under the original title: "Transplantations of Ectopic Pregnancy from Fallopian Tube to Cavity of Uterus". The article describes the procedure and reports a subsequent successful birth. An anecdote about another such transfer has been reported in other articles. The source of the anecdote was a 1990 letter to the editor of a scientific journal, but 34 years later the journal published an "Expression of Concern" about the reliability of the account described in the letter (AGOG, 2024). Based on the lack of evidence of a repeatable procedure, notwithstanding the century-old Wallace report and the 1990 letter to the editor, other sources (e.g., Thomas, 2023; Cleveland Clinic, 2020) come to the same conclusion as Ben David: the technology to accomplish this sort of transfer does not currently exist, at least not in a repeatable way.

Miscarriage

The last complication of pregnancy that I would like to briefly address is the miscarriage. As defined in Chapter 7, a miscarriage is the spontaneous natural termination of a pregnancy resulting in the loss of an embryo or fetus from the uterus during the first 20 weeks of gestational age.

I was informed that prior to the 1960s it was common practice in Catholic hospitals to baptize an embryo or fetus immediately if a miscarriage occurred (D. Bouchard, personal communication, 24 August 2025). The procedure is similar to the one described for the diseased uterus above. The interested reader may refer to Rosshirt (1959) It seems that few lay Catholics knew about this after the 1950s. However, Canon 871 in the 1983 Code of Canon Law (CIC, 1998) does indicate that this discipline is still in force: "If aborted fetuses are alive, they are to be baptized insofar as possible". Given the generality of usage of the term "abortion" outside of this treatise, this canon intends to include all cases of the loss of an unborn child, be it natural (miscarriage) or the result of a medical procedure (to include induced abortion).

During a 29 January 2025 Senate Finance Committee confirmation hearing, Senator Catherine Cortez Masto asked Robert F. Kennedy Jr. if a woman undergoing life-threatening bleeding due to an "incomplete miscarriage" has a legal right to an "emergency abortion" (Seeman, 2025). Not being an obstetrician or a woman who had experienced an incomplete miscarriage, Mr. Kennedy did not know how to respond to the question. An incomplete miscarriage is defined as a type of miscarriage in which some of the products of conception remain in the uterus, while the other products are expelled (Redinger, 2024). Senator Masto was confusing the medical procedure that removes the unexpelled products of conception with the procedure of an induced abortion. Senator Masto's question seems to display either intentional deception or an unexpected ignorance. I do not see how the removal of unexpelled products of conception can be classified as an abortion because of the lack of intent to remove a living embryo or fetus from the uterus and I assume because a living embryo or fetus does not remain in the uterus after some parts of it are expelled.

Doubts About the Origin of Human Life

Two of the greatest doubts in the debate about the origin of human life in the here and now are these:

1. The definition of a *human person*.
2. The moment at which God infuses a human soul into a human body.

A philosophical definition of the beginning of a particular human life is the point before which this particular person did not exist. This point is called *conception* or fertilization. A scientific definition of conception can be found on the website of the American College of Pediatricians (Miranda, 2017):

> The predominance of human biological research confirms that human life begins at conception—fertilization.

Pope John Paul II (1995) cites the Catholic Church's *Declaration on Procured Abortion* to explain how the Church understands the beginning of a particular human life (Sacred Congregation for the Doctrine of the Faith, 1974):

> In reality, respect for human life is called for from the time that the process of generation begins. From the time that the ovum is fertilized, a life is begun which is neither that of the father nor of the mother, it is rather the life of a new human being with his own growth. It would never be made human if it were not human already. To this perpetual evidence...modern genetic science brings valuable confirmation. It has demonstrated that, from the first instant, there is established the program of what this living being will be: a man, this individual man with his characteristic aspects already well determined. Right from fertilization is begun the adventure of a human life, and each of its capacities requires time—a rather lengthy time—to find its place and to be in a position to act.

Does a *human life* begin its existence as a *human person* (a human being of body and soul created by God) at the moment of conception, or does a human person begin its existence sometime after the conception of a human life? The answer to this question in the mind of true religion depends on exactly when God infuses a human soul into a human embryo or fetus. Biblical theology sheds light on this question in many ways. Examples can include the following from the NAB translation:

Before I formed you in the womb I knew you, before you were born I dedicated you. [Jeremiah 1:5]

When Elizabeth heard Mary's greeting, the infant leaped in her womb. [Luke 1:41]

For you drew me forth from the womb. [Psalm 22:9]

...he was named Jesus, the name given him by the angel before he was conceived in the womb. [Luke 2:21]

This biblical evidence reinforces belief that a human person exists prior to birth, while in the womb. Someone may ask the question: "Why do I care what an ancient book of myths says about anything? I don't believe in the Bible or in the Bible's God." That's a fair question, even if it makes assumptions that are unprovable. For example, archeology and independent historical accounts verify the accuracy of certain of the historical claims made in the Bible. Additionally, it is not irrational to assume that a God of Christians would make His will known to His creation, man. If a person decides to honestly and deliberately search for God, his search in many cases will demonstrate with reasonable certainty that God *must* exist. The principal task if this point is reached is to learn about this God and to seek to discover His will for His creatures. This endeavor will lead the person to discover or take more seriously religion as the jumping off point for advancement towards belief and trust in this God. With time, there may develop a desire to decide which among the plethora of religions is most likely, most certain, and most aligned with reason and reality. A somewhat in-depth study of history can assist greatly in the task of finding true religion.

The question may be asked again: at what point in time does human life become a human person? This question introduces us once again to *doubt*. Does anyone know at what point in pregnancy God infuses a soul into an unborn human life? Can it be measured or otherwise observed? Rational philosophy and speculative theology can provide reasons to assume that the human soul is infused into the human body at conception, but God alone knows with certainty the answer to this question. How are we, as individuals and society, to respond? Are we morally free to remove and dispose of an unborn child 10 seconds after conception? 10 minutes? 24 hours? 9 days? 9 weeks? 9 months? No. We are to follow the traditional code of physicians to "do no harm". But how do we know if we will be causing harm to the unborn human life by ending it before God infuses the soul? Independent of inferences from biblical evidence such as we see above, we do not and cannot know with absolute certitude at what point from conception onward God infuses the soul into the body, for public revelation ceased nearly two millennia ago, and a definitive answer to the specific question of the moment of infusion was not given by Christ or the Apostles before public revelation ended. This condition of unknowing is a condition of doubt. How do we resolve our doubt? We cannot resolve our doubt without a definitive answer from our Creator, but we can choose the most *prudent* path, which is to *assume* that the soul could be infused into a human life at the start of an individual human existence, meaning *at conception*. In concrete terms, the only way to be *absolutely certain* of doing no harm is to refrain from aborting an unborn child at every stage of development, from conception to natural birth. The *Declaration on Procured Abortion* (Sacred Congregation for the Doctrine of the Faith, 1974) puts it this way (emphasis mine):

> *It is a philosophical problem from which our moral affirmation remains independent* for two reasons: (1) supposing a belated animation, there is still nothing less than a human life, preparing for and calling for a soul in which the nature received from parents is completed; (2) on the other hand, *it suffices that this presence of the soul be probable (and one can never prove the contrary)* in order that the taking of life involve accepting the risk of killing a man, not only waiting for, but already in possession of his soul.

The instruction *Dignitas Personae* was cited in Chapter 7 as support for the proposition that an embryo conceived in a laboratory is indeed a human person. I cite it again here to demonstrate that the Catholic understanding that life begins at conception is not based on authority alone, but also on reason. From *Dignitas Personae* (Sacred Congregation for the Doctrine of the Faith, 2008), emphasis: mine:

> *Although the presence of the spiritual soul cannot be observed experimentally, the conclusions of science regarding the human embryo give "a valuable indication for discerning by the use of reason* a personal presence at the moment of

> the first appearance of a human life: how could a human individual not be a human person?".

Thus, those are in error who would argue that Catholicism merely *asserts on the basis of authority alone* that the life of a human person begins at conception. In my opinion, the Catholic understanding that the totality of the human person logically must *in a moral sense* exist from conception onward is based as much on reason and prudence as on authority by itself. *Dignitas Personae* says this about the human person (Sacred Congregation for the Doctrine of the Faith, 2008):

> Thus the fruit of human generation, from the first moment of its existence, that is to say from the moment the zygote has formed, demands the unconditional respect that is morally due to the human being in his bodily and spiritual totality. The human being is to be respected and treated as a person from the moment of conception; and therefore from that same moment his rights as a person must be recognized, among which in the first place is the inviolable right of every innocent human being to life.

On the basis of a declaration from the 4th Lateran Council and Pope Pius XII's insistence in *Humani Generis* (Pope Pius XII, 1950) that God created the first man, Fr. Ott in his *Fundamentals of Catholic Dogma* (1960) considers the creation of the first man by God a *de fide* doctrine, in other words, a dogma. For those who accept this doctrine, and those who accept the theological conclusion that the first woman was in some way derived from the first man, the immediate infusion of a human soul at the beginning of the existence (i.e., the "conception") of Adam and Eve (as described in Chapter 6) may serve as a parallel to the time at which a human soul is infused into a preborn child: at the moment of the person's creation. For all who were born after Adam and Eve, their creation occurs at their conception.

For Catholic readers, there is another dogma that concerns the origin of a human person: the dogma of the *Immaculate Conception.* My bioethicist colleague, Fr. Benedict, suggested in early 2025 (personal communication, 24 April 2025) that this dogma strengthens adherence to the belief that the human soul is infused at conception. This dogma assumes that the first sin of Adam (defined as the *original sin*) produced negative results for the human person, among these being the loss of sanctifying grace, infused knowledge, bodily immortality, the beatific vision in the next life, and freedom from concupiscence. The dogma tells us that Jesus' mother Mary, as a human person with body and soul, was preserved at conception from the privation of sanctifying grace. Since only a human person can suffer from this affliction, preservation from it at conception assumes that the human personhood of Mary began at conception.

Let us give further consideration, for a moment, to the Catholic dogma of the Immaculate Conception. This dogma is predicated on another dogma equally binding on Catholics: the dogma of "original sin". The dogma of original sin states that all men are born in a condition of privation of sanctifying grace due to the first sin of Adam. This condition in human persons is referred to as existence in a *state of original sin.* The negative effects of Adam's first sin are believed to be passed down by human procreation to every human person that ever existed and ever will exist in the present age of mankind, with the exception of Jesus Christ and His mother. Original sin is considered in Catholic theology to be a *wound* on man's nature; it is not a destruction of human nature, but a wound (also considered a "stain" on the soul) that can be healed through baptism (see the Glossary). Here is the definition of the Immaculate Conception (Pope Pius IX, 1854):

> We declare, pronounce, and define that the doctrine which holds that the most Blessed Virgin Mary, in the first instance of her conception, by a singular grace and privilege granted by Almighty God, in view of the merits of Jesus Christ, the Savior of the human race, was preserved free from all stain of original sin, is a doctrine revealed by God and therefore to be believed firmly and constantly by all the faithful.

On consideration of the precise wording of this dogmatic definition, it is seen that a *singular* grace and privilege was granted by God to Mary at *her* conception. As suggested above by Fr. Benedict, it could be reasoned from this definition that since Mary came into existence as a human person at the moment of her conception, by the logic of induction all human beings come into existence as human persons at the moment of their conception. This may, however, be a weak argument because the infusion of Mary's soul at conception could also have been a singular privilege granted to her alone.

I stumbled upon a book online recently that attempted to defend a woman's "right to choose". One of the arguments cited by the author reveals a lot about the misapprehension of the abortionist: homicide has rights when it supports a person's convenience. The claim is that even if society and the courts were to acknowledge that an unborn child is a human *and* legal person, the homicide of the unborn child is justice because the child did not get the mother's permission to be inside of her, to steal her nutrients, and to cause her discomfort and inconvenience. This is the inverse of the position I have been discussing with colleagues for years:

> The abortionist must have the permission of the unborn child before the abortion homicide (or "assisted suicide" if the child would agree to be killed) could even be considered.

The abortionist's argument, as nearly always, embraces the wrong moral object. The correct moral object in all *abortions proper* is the right to life of the *innocent* unborn child. The proper moral object is not the inconvenience and discomfort of the mother, who could have avoided the trauma by simply abstaining from sexual relations, or in the case of rape, by offering her suffering up to God in joy that God has blessed her with the opportunity to bring a new human life into the world.

My tone in the two paragraphs above may come across as rude, uncaring, or imprecise. If so, I apologize for what may appear as bluntness. I would like to quote a more eloquent articulation from a former prefect of the Congregation for the Doctrine of the Faith (now called "Dicastery"), Cardinal Gerhard Müller, who recently spoke in defense of the unborn. Here is the portion of his message relevant to the moral object in questions about pregnancy and the right to life of the unborn (Müller, 2025):

> The human being who is born is the same person who was carried under his mother's heart for nine months and who was conceived by his parents physically. ...Weighing the mother's right to self-determination against her child's right to life...obscures the truth that one person's right to self-determination ends where another person's right to life begins. ...The child's right to life is far more important than the parents' right to self-determination. We must think from the perspective of the child's life and not from the needs and interests of those who stand in his way and violently take his life. The right to self-determination is about freedom from external control, which I must also grant to others. Children are entrusted to their parents for the purpose of education. Parents, however, are not masters of the life and death of their own children.

CHAPTER 10

WORDS MEAN THINGS

The Dignity of One Human Life

The message of this treatise is offered from the perspective of the temporal and eternal dignity of one human life. The message is this: human life is precious both to man and to God. This is the Catholic perspective, and it is shared by other religions and ecclesial bodies. The human life of primary concern here is that of born and unborn children. I begin with born children. In the first months of life a child is for the most part useless in terms of utility. However, this child is useful in terms of sharing. This child can share its mother's and father's lives, the lives of its brothers and sisters, even the lives of its extended family members. The child, when the privation of habitual grace is eliminated, can share with people of all ages and states in life a human participation in the internal life of God. As pointed out in Chapter 8, this participation is a gift freely given by God to all who do not oppose, but who respond in acceptance to, God's sanctifying grace, which is always available to those who, with a pure heart, ask for it.

The human person was first created with the proximate purpose of sharing in the life of God by knowing, loving, and serving Him in this life. After paradise was lost, a remote purpose for the life of a human person was added to this. This purpose is to be happy with God for all eternity in knowledge, love, and service to Him in the afterlife. To know, love, and serve God is a responsibility that must not be shirked by anyone. There are many who reject this charge, but there are as well many who accept and act on it. It would be prudent for those who reject their responsibility to God to reconsider, as Pascal did, what this rejection can result in for the human soul: the possibility of loss of nearness to God for eternity after death.

The Three "Exceptions"

As mentioned in previous chapters, it seems necessary to me that in order to advance the pro-life cause, inaccurate and imprecise terms must be discarded, and new, more accurate and precise terms must be developed. Why? Because of the ubiquitous misconceptions of certain highly educated and lesser educated people about what is and is not an abortion, what is and is not a human person, what is or is not man's obligation to the protection and preservation of human life before God. For example, apparently well-meaning politicians and practitioners of religion of all stripes declare: "Abortion should be impermissible in all cases, ***except***..." Here is where they name their poison: "cases of *rape*, *incest*, or threat to *the life of the mother*". Each of these common "exceptions" must be examined.

The *first exception* is usually "rape". What is rape? Rape is the forced sexual violation of a person by a vicious criminal. Who is responsible for a rape? Answer: the criminal who assaulted the innocent victim. Who are the victim(s) of a rape? Answer: the one assaulted and the new human life if the assault resulted in the unwanted pregnancy of a female victim. Who is to pay restitution for the assault? Answer: the criminal who committed crime. Who is to suffer the potentially longer-lasting consequences of the assault? Answer: the victim and any new life that may have resulted from the assault. How is the victim and any new child to recover from the assault? Well, this is where the confusion usually begins. In the mind of the person improperly trained in morality (i.e., ethics, with God as the absolute arbiter of right and wrong), and in the mind of malicious persons, it often happens that the moral object of the pregnancy is misplaced onto the convenience (or as Cardinal Müller says, the self-determination) of the mother. But, as described in Chapter 9, this is the wrong moral object. Two (or more) actual lives matter here: the mother and the unborn child. The mother suffered physical, emotional, and even spiritual harm from the assault. Would a judge declare that she deserves to die, perhaps for not suffering enough? No, because that would constitute a severe injustice. What about the other life, that of the unborn child (or children, if twins)? Does this person deserve to die because he has not suffered enough, because he is tiny and defenseless, because he is guilty of committing a crime against his mother? No, because that would constitute a severe injustice against the child. But, you may ask, what about the inconvenience of the mother? Will she not have to change her future plans, her lifestyle, perhaps her means of support or even where she lives? Perhaps she will, but there are other options, options which have served people well for millennia: (1) care for the born child by a family member or close friend, (2) adoption, (3) foster care, (4) perhaps others. But, you may ask, are these not inconveniences that interfere with the life the mother had planned on living? Are these not additional burdens that she will have to reckon with? Is it "fair" to consider the life of the unborn child ahead of the convenience of the mother, who is likely a person capable of caring for the child, capable of earning a living, capable of living a married life, capable of turning to family for assistance?

It has often been said that life is not fair. I suppose a non-Christian or a young person can believe this, but a mature Christian cannot. For a mature Christian, the burdens of life represent an opportunity, an opportunity to offer up one's sufferings to God. Supporting evidence is found in the Bible. From Colossians 1:24 in the NAB:

> Now I rejoice in my sufferings for your sake, and in my flesh I am filling up what is lacking in the afflictions of Christ on behalf of his body, which is the Church.

From Romans 5:3-4 in the NAB:

> ...we even boast of our afflictions, knowing that affliction produces endurance, and endurance, proven character, and proven character, hope.

Thus, instead of being beaten down, demoralized, or thrown into depression by affliction, a Christian ought to consider it a door opening, a door through which the Christian is able to join his own suffering to the afflictions that Christ suffered long ago on the wood of the tree, but which are still efficacious for the one who reaches out to Him today.

The *second exception* is incest. There are valid moral and practical reasons for considering incest an undesirable act after the age of the first generations of mankind. I see no need to list these. I will merely point out that the moral object remains the same as in the case of rape: the life of the mother and the protection and preservation of the life of the unborn child are paramount.

The *third exception* is a threat to the life of the woman. This situation was discussed in Chapter 9 and can constitute a moral challenge with a known remedy. In this circumstance, the quality of the medical system becomes critical for both the woman and the unborn child within her. A rational and morally-legitimate medical system would never consider subjecting the woman to an induced abortion, due to the nature of this crime. On the other hand, when the moral constraints discussed Chapter 9 are taken into consideration, a medical procedure may have to be performed to save the life of the woman, while knowing that the unborn child will not survive the procedure.

Elephant in the Room – A Fourth "Exception"?

During the SARS-CoV-2 assault against the healthy, the Catholic Church made perhaps one of the most cowardly decisions in its two-millennial history: this Church acquiesced to the cessation of administration of the Sacraments in the face of a threat of disease and possible death induced by what appears to me to be a biological weapon. There were numerous ways the Church could have responded short of cutting off access to the remedies for spiritual illness and death. In my own way, I tried to lead the local Church in some of these ways. For example, I sent my archdiocese a plan for holding the Sacraments outdoors (among the safest environments possible), a plan that was compatible with the secular guidelines for safe distancing between individuals in closed environments. For the entire academic year, I held the class that I was teaching outdoors, except for one extremely cold Sunday. I increased ventilation in all classrooms and spaced individuals according to Archdiocesan and CDC (U.S. Centers for Disease Control) guidelines. I installed a sound system in my parish gymnasium so that Mass could be offered in a larger facility where safe spacing could be arranged according to the guidelines mentioned above.

When I say that being outdoors was among the safest environments possible during the Covid pandemic, I am speaking as an atmospheric scientist and health physicist. On a typical morning the planetary boundary layer (lowest layer of the earth's daytime and usually night-time atmosphere) rises with the rising sun. It is known that the most efficient transfer of airborne contaminants takes place by turbulent advection. In the case of the rising boundary layer, the turbulence is primarily in the vertical direction as turbulent convection. The turbulent convection both carries upward and diffuses away whatever contaminants are exhaled by persons on the ground; e.g., viruses and the larger aerosols to which they adhere. This turbulent dispersion acts in concert with N95, similar respirators, and even surgical and layered-cloth masks to reduce the concentration of viruses and aerosols that protected individuals inhale. Under the circumstances of outdoor activities and the taking of simple precautions, it would not be especially easy to inhale a viral load sufficient to cause infection by SARS-Cov-2.

Thus, holding activities such as Catholic Mass, Sacraments, and instruction outdoors is a way to safely accommodate large gatherings during threats such as the SARS-CoV-2 assault. I consider it a crime against faith that many religious leaders allowed themselves to remain so ignorant of basic science during the assault, especially when they had recourse to parishioners with the expertise and offer of assistance needed to conduct liturgies in a safe manner. St. Augustine's warning comes to mind.

Regarding "vaccination" against the Covid-19 disease, guidance was offered by the Congregation for the Doctrine of the Faith (CDF) about how a Catholic was to react to the "vaccines" that were released in late 2020, especially since the "vaccines" legally available in the United States were either tested with recourse to children killed by elective abortion or actually incorporated abortion-derived material during the production process (Update, 2021). In a doctrinal note issued on 21 December 2020, the CDF stated: "it is morally acceptable to receive Covid-19 vaccines that have used cell lines from aborted fetuses in their research and production process" (Sacred Congregation for the Doctrine of the Faith, 2020). The rationale underlying this statement is revealing:

> The fundamental reason for considering the use of these vaccines morally licit is that the kind of cooperation in evil (passive material cooperation) in the procured abortion from which these cell lines originate is, on the part of those making use of the resulting vaccines, remote.

One man's cure is another man's poison. Remote, passive, and material cooperation with evil, no matter how it is offered up, remains cooperation with evil. To its credit, the CDF qualified its opinion above in the same doctrinal note:

> At the same time, practical reason makes evident that vaccination is not, as a rule, a moral obligation and that, therefore, it must be voluntary.

The doctrinal note went on to explain the precautions needed to be taken by those who refuse to cooperate in any way with the evil of abortion. This refusal is the pro-life position. The recommendation of the doctrinal note was practical and not all that difficult to do:

> Those who, however, for reasons of conscience, refuse vaccines produced with cell lines from aborted fetuses, must do their utmost to avoid, by other prophylactic means and appropriate behavior, becoming vehicles for the transmission of the infectious agent.

Everyone learned a few months later, however, that the "vaccines" produced without sufficient testing and precautions were ineffective at preventing the transmission of the disease. Given that by this time natural immunity had already begun to take effect, and the fact that other strains of the virus had displaced the earlier one, "vaccination" became a merely speculative remedy for the illness.

The question then asked by the faithful Catholic mind was the following:

> Why would a person choose to cooperate with the evil of abortion (reception of a "vaccine" injection) when the products of this evil (the "vaccine") were ineffective at accomplishing what they were intended to do?

The pro-life position was the right one all along.

Justification for Recognizing the Value of Preborn Human Life

In Chapter 2, I proposed a change in medical terminology related to pregnancy and complications of pregnancy. I then spent many pages explaining the Christian, predominantly Catholic, basis for the moral value of preborn human life. This basis is primarily theological and philosophical. The justification for the protection and preservation of human life, especially the most innocent among us, cannot be convincingly argued from an atheistic materialist perspective (as defined in Chapter 4) because this perspective is purely relativistic, physicalist, and totally without a reason for hope in a rational vision of justice and happiness in an afterlife. Without hope for a better afterlife than can be achieved in temporal life in this world, the atheistic materialist must seek out as much comfort, pleasure, and relative security as he is able to acquire. Because of finite human nature, the atheistic materialist's physical satisfactions can never be completely fulfilled. This is due to the fact that there is more to human existence than this life, than this world; there is the opportunity for absolute and eternal satisfaction and fulfillment in the afterlife. If there were no actual afterlife, human life in this world could have no value beyond the sentimental, the transient, the forgotten. Thus, the justification for recognizing the value of preborn human life is that God assigns value to this life.

An Attempt at New Definitions

For the reasons given in Chapter 3, I believe that a revision in presentation of pro-life principles is needed and must begin with a redefinition of select elements of the terminology relevant to abortion, medical afflictions and procedures, and obstacles to a successful pregnancy and delivery. I think that the task of redefinition can be most fruitful if the lexicon to be used predates the current linguistic anarchy in English and the current degeneration of sexual morality. Therefore, just as in the opening sections of Chapter 3, I advocate that inaccurate and imprecise terminology be jettisoned and that more descriptive and accurate terminology be constructed to replace it. As a nonspecialist in the medical and public health fields, what I am proposing is only a start, an example, an advocacy for a revised approach to the discourse on the pro-life cause that makes more precise the labels attached to medical conditions and procedures in accordance with the nature of the conditions and the function of the procedures used to treat these conditions. I call upon medical and health professionals to join me in this endeavor with their expertise.

In Chapter 9, I briefly examined two types of complications of pregnancy: one was a complication due to a preexisting medical condition, while the other was a complication due to the nature of the pregnancy itself. I also listed five other ectopic complications of pregnancy, and the complication known as miscarriage. I spoke about the proper Catholic response to miscarriage and gave an example of an incorrect response by a politician to a case of an incomplete miscarriage. It is in cases such as these that proper terminology is most important. According to my proposed definition of abortion (the direct termination of a pregnancy, from conception to birth, with the intent to destroy a human life), the removal of any unexpelled products of conception does not represent the termination of a pregnancy, since the incomplete miscarriage has already accomplished that, but does represent a medical procedure to restore the health of the woman for whom her pregnancy unintentionally ended. These procedures have names such as "expectant management", "pharmaceutical treatment", and "surgical treatment". None of these procedures should be considered an abortion.

Hydatidiform moles are often called molar pregnancies. In a *complete hydatidiform mole* (see the glossary) an embryo cannot form and is thus not a pregnancy (Cleveland Clinic, 2022). It should therefore not be referred to as a pregnancy. *Partial hydatidiform moles* can be referred to as complications of pregnancy that up until the year 2022 had produced 13 documented live births of children who lived more than 30 days (Walsh, 2022).

A Secular Justification for a More Accurate Redefinition of Medical Terms Related to Abortion

I recently realized another argument that favors the redefinition of medical terms related to abortion. According to a news item posted not long ago on YouTube, a woman was "denied a necessary abortion in Texas after its ban" (YouTube, 2025). Was she really denied an abortion? Not according to my advocacy for a redefinition of certain medical terms. You see, the woman was the victim of a Fallopian-tube implantation. It was reported that during her ectopic pregnancy, her Fallopian tube ruptured, whereupon she required emergency surgery to remove the ruptured tube in order to make sure her life would be out of jeopardy. Her complaint after the surgery was that prior to the rupture she was sent home to potentially die. Could her physician have been morally justified in removing the tube earlier in the pregnancy before it had ruptured? Healy (1963) speaks in detail about exactly this type of situation in his book on medical ethics, an excerpt of which appears on the EWTN website (Healy, 2025). He points out that once the embryo implants in the Fallopian tube, it begins to damage the tube wall as it seeks nourishment. If left untreated, the progress of this damage could eventually lead to the rupture the woman eventually suffered from. Healy says that if monitoring by her physician would have revealed that the damage to the tube had become sufficiently advanced, her physician would have been morally justified in removing the pathological tube before it had a chance to rupture and place the woman's life at even greater risk of death. It seems likely that the woman needed surgical intervention prior to the rupture in order to treat this potentially life-threatening complication of pregnancy. As explained in Chapter 9, the intention of the surgery would not be to abort her unborn child, but to save her life. Her situation was a first-class example of the principle of double effect in action. In Chapter 9 I referred to the surgery that she probably should have received earlier in her pregnancy as a *tubal therapeutic excision with child.* The exact labeling is not important. What is important is that the excision would not directly attack the child, but would remove the tube that the child sadly existed inside of. The mother would live as a result of the procedure, but the child would die as an unintended consequence.

I checked the Texas Health and Safety Code (Title 4.B, Section 245.002) and found that an act that causes the death of an unborn child of a pregnant woman is not considered an abortion if the intent of the act is to remove an ectopic pregnancy (Texas Statute, 1989). This acknowledgment is quite meritorious. However, even though the removal of an ectopic pregnancy is considered a legitimate medical treatment by the Texas Code (Texas Amended Statute, 2025), particularly in situations where the woman's life is threatened by this complication of pregnancy, the Code as written and implemented still raises two causes for concern: (1) the manner of removal of the ectopic pregnancy is not specified (e.g., the removal could happen by direct chemical or surgical attack on the unborn child), and (2) the law is evidently not widely known by not only the general public, but perhaps even by medical personnel as well.

Conclusion

This treatise is an attempt to improve the presentation of pro-life principles in order to make them more understandable and rational to the reader who rejects the current arguments in favor of life, as well as to those who accept the existing arguments, but who do not articulate well their basis for accepting them. Given the war waged against reason and true religion in schools, universities, the popular media, the military, and currently many government and non-governmental institutions in the country, not to mention the ubiquitous political sophistry, a clear and convincing pro-life message must be promoted by those not blinded or cowed by the current levers of power. A dark age has embarked against the good, the true, and the beautiful. This time the assault is against innocence, the truth about the human person as body and soul created by God, and human life itself. It is time to fight back with the best tools, the best arguments, and the best religion.

APPENDIX

Excerpt from the Athanasian Creed that Bears on the Nature of the Trinity and the Incarnation

...And the Catholic Faith is this, that we worship one God in Trinity and Trinity in Unity. Neither confounding the Persons, nor dividing the Substance. For there is one Person of the Father, another of the Son, and another of the Holy Ghost. But the Godhead of the Father, of the Son and of the Holy Ghost is all One, the Glory Equal, the Majesty Co-Eternal. Such as the Father is, such is the Son, and such is the Holy Ghost. The Father Uncreate[d], the Son Uncreate[d], and the Holy Ghost Uncreate[d]. The Father Incomprehensible, the Son Incomprehensible, and the Holy Ghost Incomprehensible. The Father Eternal, the Son Eternal, and the Holy Ghost Eternal and yet they are not Three Eternals but One Eternal. As also there are not Three Uncreated, nor Three Incomprehensibles, but One Uncreated, and One Incomprehensible. So likewise the Father is Almighty, the Son Almighty, and the Holy Ghost Almighty. And yet they are not Three Almighties but One Almighty.

So the Father is God, the Son is God, and the Holy Ghost is God. And yet they are not Three Gods, but One God. So likewise the Father is Lord, the Son Lord, and the Holy Ghost Lord. And yet not Three Lords but One Lord. For, like as we are compelled by the Christian verity to acknowledge every Person by Himself to be God and Lord, so are we forbidden by the Catholic Religion to say, there be Three Gods or Three Lords. The Father is made of none, neither created, nor begotten. The Son is of the Father alone; not made, nor created, but begotten. The Holy Ghost is of the Father, and of the Son neither made, nor created, nor begotten, but proceeding.

So there is One Father, not Three Fathers; one Son, not Three Sons; One Holy Ghost, not Three Holy Ghosts. And in this Trinity none is afore or after Other, None is greater or less than Another, but the whole Three Persons are Co-eternal together, and Co-equal. So that in all things, as is aforesaid, the Unity in Trinity, and the Trinity in Unity, is to be worshipped. He therefore that will be saved, must thus think of the Trinity.

Furthermore, it is necessary to everlasting Salvation, that he also believe rightly the Incarnation of our Lord Jesus Christ. For the right Faith is, that we believe and confess, that our Lord Jesus Christ, the Son of God, is God and Man.

God, of the substance of the Father, begotten before the worlds; and Man, of the substance of His mother, born into the world. Perfect God and Perfect Man, of a reasonable Soul and human Flesh subsisting. Equal to the Father as touching His Godhead, and inferior to the Father as touching His Manhood. Who, although He be God and Man, yet He is not two, but One Christ. One, not by conversion of the Godhead into Flesh, but by taking of the Manhood into God. One altogether, not by confusion of substance, but by Unity of Person. For as the reasonable soul and flesh is one Man, so God and Man is one Christ…

REFERENCES

AS CITED IN THE CHAPTERS

Chapter 2

Catechisim of the Catholic Church (November 2019). 2nd edition. United States Conference of Catholic Bishops. Nos. 293-294. https://www.usccb.org/sites/default/files/flipbooks/catechism/78/

CIC (1998). *Code of Canon Law: Latin-English Edition*. Translated by the Canon Law Society of America. Pp. 279-280. See also: https://www.vatican.va/archive/cod-iuris-canonici/eng/documents/cic_lib4-cann834-878_en.html

Greek Medicine: The Hippocratic Oath (2002). Courtesy of the National Library of Medicine. https://www.nlm.nih.gov/hmd/greek/greek_oath.html

Hardon, John A. (1980). *Modern Catholic Dictionary*. Doubleday. Garden City, New York. P. 171.

Ott, Ludwig (May 1960). *Fundamentals of Catholic Dogma*. 4th edition. TAN Books, Rockford, Illinois. Pp. 4-10.

Pope Leo XIV (4 October 2025). *Dilexi Te*. Apostolic exhortation. https://www.vatican.va/content/leo-xiv/en/apost_exhortations/documents/20251004-dilexi-te.html

Pope Paul VI (21 November 1964). *Lumen Gentium: Dogmatic Constitution on The Church*. Second Vatican Council. No. 16. https://www.vatican.va/archive/hist_councils/ii_vatican_council/documents/vat-ii_const_19641121_lumen-gentium_en.html

Pope Paul VI (18 November 1965). *Dei Verbum: Dogmatic Constitution on Divine Revelation.* Second Vatican Council. Nos. 7-8, 15-17.
https://www.vatican.va/archive/hist_councils/ii_vatican_council/documents/vat-ii_const_19651118_dei-verbum_en.html

Pope Paul VI (30 June 1968). *Solemni Hac Liturgia* (*Credo of the People of God*). No. 23. https://www.vatican.va/content/paul-vi/en/motu_proprio/documents/hf_p-vi_motu-proprio_19680630_credo.html

Sacred Congregation for the Doctrine of the Faith (24 May 1990). *Donum Veritatis.* Nos. 13-17.
https://www.vatican.va/roman_curia/congregations/cfaith/documents/rc_con_cfaith_doc_19900524_theologian-vocation_en.html

Slater, Thomas (1910). Moral Aspect of Divine Law. In *The Catholic Encyclopedia.* Robert Appleton Company. New York.
https://www.newadvent.org/cathen/09071a.htm

Steinsaltz, Adin (15 October 2017). *Koren Talmud Bavli: Noe Edition.* Volume 31: Makkot Shevuot. The William Davidson digital edition.
https://www.sefaria.org/Makkot.23b.18?lang=bi&with=all&lang2=en

Chapter 3

Dodds, Io (19 April 2023). Meet the Elite Couples Breeding to Save Mankind. *The Telegraph.*

https://www.telegraph.co.uk/family/life/pronatalists-save-mankind-by-having-babies-silicon-valley/

Mahdawi, Arwa (21 April 2023). "Hipster Eugenics": Why is the Media Cosying Up to People Who Want to Build a Super Race? *The Guardian*. https://www.theguardian.com/lifeandstyle/2023/apr/20/pro-natalism-babies-global-population-genetics

Pope John Paul II (25 March 1995). *Evangelium Vitae*. No. 62. https://www.vatican.va/content/john-paul-ii/en/encyclicals/documents/hf_jp-ii_enc_25031995_evangelium-vitae.html

Pope Paul VI (7 December 1965a). *Gaudium et Spes: Pastoral Constitution on the Church in the Modern World*. Second Vatican Council. No. 27. https://www.vatican.va/archive/hist_councils/ii_vatican_council/documents/vat-ii_const_19651207_gaudium-et-spes_en.html

Pope Paul VI (7 December 1965b). *Dignitatis Humanae: Declaration on Religious Freedom*. Second Vatican Council. No. 1. https://www.vatican.va/archive/hist_councils/ii_vatican_council/documents/vat-ii_decl_19651207_dignitatis-humanae_en.html

Porter, Tom (19 April 2023). Elon Musk and Tucker Carlson Discussed the Urge to Have Sex, with Musk Claiming "Birth Control and Abortions" Could Cause Civilization to Collapse. *Business Insider*. https://www.businessinsider.com/elon-musk-tucker-carlson-sex-procreation-collapse-civilisation-abortion-pill-2023-4?op=1

YouTube podcast (31 December 2025). Posted by Katie Halper. https://www.youtube.com/watch?v=FV_naFC1r78

Chapter 4

Boethius (circa 520). *Liber De Persona et Duabus Naturis Contra Eutychen Et Nestorium.* Chapter III. Courtesy of biblehub.com. https://biblehub.com/library/boethius/the_theological_tractates/a_treatise_against_eutyches_and.htm#1

Kirby, Peter (2023). "The Didache". *Early Christian Writings.* http://www.earlychristianwritings.com/text/didache-roberts.html

Pascal, Blaise (collection of notes first published posthumously in 1670). https://www.gutenberg.org/files/18269/18269-h/18269-h.htm

Pope John Paul II (25 March 1995). *Evangelium Vitae.* No. 2. https://www.vatican.va/content/john-paul-ii/en/encyclicals/documents/hf_jp-ii_enc_25031995_evangelium-vitae.html

Slater, Thomas (1910). Justice. In *The Catholic Encyclopedia.* Robert Appleton Company. New York. http://www.newadvent.org/cathen/08571c.htm

Chapter 5

Augustine of Hippo (A.D. 415). *The Literal Meaning of Genesis* (*De Genesi ad Literam*). In the Ancient Christian Writers series, No. 41 (1982). Paulist Press. Mahwah, NJ. Pp. 42-43.

Bates, Sarah A. (11 May 2025). *Deoxyribonucleic Acid (DNA)*. Public domain. National Human Genome Research Institute. https://www.genome.gov/genetics-glossary/Deoxyribonucleic-Acid-DNA

Blount, Zarchary D., Richard E. Lenski, Jonathan B. Losos (9 November 2018). Contingency and Determinism in Evolution: Replaying Life's Tape *Science*. **362**(6415). DOI: 10.1126/science.aam5979. https://www.science.org/doi/10.1126/science.aam5979

Chatterjee, Nimrat, Graham C. Walker (June 2017). Mechanisms of DNA Damage, Repair and Mutagenesis. *Environ Mol Mutagen*. **58**(5): 235–263. Published online 9 May 2017 at DOI: 10.1002/em.22087. https://www.ncbi.nlm.nih.gov/pmc/articles/PMC5474181/

Fitzgerald, Devon M., Susan M. Rosenberg (1 April 2019). What is Mutation? A Chapter in the Series: How Microbes "Jeopardize" the Modern Synthesis. *PLOS Genetics*. **15**(4): e1007995. https://doi.org/10.1371/journal.pgen.1007995

Liao, Shijun, Shijie Qin (25 April 2025). Noise-Expansion Cascade: An Origin of Randomness of Turbulence. *Journal of Fluid Mechanics*. **1009**(A2). doi:10.1017/jfm.2025.140. https://www.cambridge.org/core/journals/journal-of-fluid-mechanics/article/noiseexpansion-cascade-an-origin-of-randomness-of-turbulence/F4FA44B1956F4D620D4CCA84C7E8B123

Luckow, Melissa (1995). Species Concepts: Assumptions, Methods, and Applications. Sytematic Botany. **20**(4): pp. 589-605. https://www.jstor.org/stable/2419812

Mas, Alix, Lagadeuc, Yvan, Vandenkoornhuyse, Philippe (27 October 2020). Reflections on the Predictability of Evolution: Toward a Conceptual Framework. *iScience*. **23**(11). DOI: 10.1016/j.isci.2020.101736. https://pmc.ncbi.nlm.nih.gov/articles/PMC7666346/

Mandock, Randal (22 March 2014): *Global Climate Change Data Through 2013*. Southern Atlantic Coast Section of the American Association of Physics Teachers Spring Meeting, Spelman College, Atlanta, Georgia.

Mandock, Randal (2016). *Introduction to Quantitative Earth Science: Beta Edition*. Linus Learning. Ronkonkoma, NY. Chapter 13.

National Academy of Sciences (2025). Definition of "evolution", under *Definitions of Evolutionary Terms*. https://www.nationalacademies.org/evolution/definitions

Russell, Sara S., Chris J. Ballentine, Monica M. Grady (17 April 2017). The Origin, History and Role of Water in the Evolution of the Early Solar System. *Philosophical Transactions of the Royal Society A*. **375**: 20170108. https://royalsocietypublishing.org/doi/10.1098/rsta.2017.0108

Spencer, Roy (7 February 2014). *95% of Climate Models Agree: The Observations Must be Wrong*. http://www.drroyspencer.com/2014/02/95-of-climate-models-agree-the-observations-must-be-wrong/

Chapter 6

Aquinas, Thomas (1274). *Summa Theologiae.* I.65-74. Online edition courtesy of Kevin Knight (2017). https://www.newadvent.org/summa/2093.htm

Bergsma, John, and Brant Pitre (2018). *A Catholic Introduction to the Bible: The Old Testament*. Ignatius Press, San Francisco. Pp. 95-97.

Pope Pius XII (12 August 1950). *Humani Generis.* No. 36. https://www.vatican.va/content/pius-xii/en/encyclicals/documents/hf_p-xii_enc_12081950_humani-generis.html

Tarbuck, Edward J., and Frederick K. Lutgens (2012). *Earth Science.* Prentice Hall. Upper Saddle River, NJ. Pp. 348-350.

Chapter 7

AAPC (2025). *Pregnancy with Abortive Outcome.* https://www.aapc.com/codes/icd-10-codes-range/O00-O9A/O00-O08/

Burbridge, Michael F. (22 January 2025). *The Christian Family, In Vitro Fertilization, and Heroic Witness to True Love.* Diocese of Arlington, Virginia. Courtesy of CatholicCulture.org. https://www.catholicculture.org/culture/library/view.cfm?recnum=12743

Christianson MS, Stern JE, Sun F, Zhang H, Styer AK, Vitek W, Polotsky AJ. Embryo cryopreservation and utilization in the United States from 2004-2013. F&S Reports 2020 Sep

28;1(2):71-77. doi: 10.1016/j.xfre.2020.05.010. https://pubmed.ncbi.nlm.nih.gov/34223221/

GA Code § 31-10-1 (2024). *2024 Code of Georgia.* Title 31, Chapter 10, Section 31-10-1. https://law.justia.com/codes/georgia/title-31/chapter-10/section-31-10-1/

Gacek (2009). Conceiving Pregnancy: U.S. Medical Dictionaries and Their Definitions of Conception and Pregnancy. *National Catholic Bioethics Quarterly.* **9**(3): 543-553. https://downloads.frc.org/EF/EF09D12.pdf

Klaus , Hannah (2025). *Reproductive Technology: Evaluation and Treatment of Infertility – Guidelines for Catholic Couples.* NFPP/US Conference of Catholic Bishops. Washington, DC: USCCB. 2025. Used with permission. https://catholicism.org/usccb-publishes-guidelines-for-catholic-couples-on-reproductive-technologies.html

Lanfranchi, Angela (20 June 2024). *What Catholic Social Teaching Says About the Status of Embryos Part One.* https://www.cathmed.org/the-pulse/what-catholic-social-teaching-says-about-the-status-of-embryos/

Medical News Today (28 June 2018). *Miscarriage: What You Need to Know.* https://www.medicalnewstoday.com/articles/262941

MedlinePlus (2 July 2025). *Miscarriage.* https://medlineplus.gov/miscarriage.html

Mirkes, Renee (28 February 2025). An Open Letter to JD Vance About IVF. *Catholic World Report.* https://www.catholicworldreport.com/2025/02/28/an-open-letter-to-jd-vance-about-ivf/

Pope John Paul II (23 May 1988). *Acta Apostolicae Sedis.* Pontifical Commission for the Authentic Interpretation of the Code of Canon Law. II.1. P. 1818. https://archive.org/details/aas-80-1988-ocr/page/1818/mode/2up

Pope John Paul II (25 March 1995). *Evangelium Vitae.* Nos. 58, 62-63. https://www.vatican.va/content/john-paul-ii/en/encyclicals/documents/hf_jp-ii_enc_25031995_evangelium-vitae.html

Sacred Congregation for the Doctrine of the Faith (22 February 1987). *Donum Vitae.* Introduction: 4-5, I.1, I.5, II.A.5, II.B.4.a, II.B.5. https://www.vatican.va/roman_curia/congregations/cfaith/documents/rc_con_cfaith_doc_19870222_respect-for-human-life_en.html

Sacred Congregation for the Doctrine of the Faith (8 September 2008). *Dignitas Personae.* Nos. 5, 16, 21-23; End note 46. https://www.vatican.va/roman_curia/congregations/cfaith/documents/rc_con_cfaith_doc_20081208_dignitas-personae_en.html

U.S. Centers for Disease Control and Prevention (26 August 2025). *About Stillbirth.* https://www.cdc.gov/stillbirth/about/index.html

Chapter 8

Augustine of Hippo (A.D. 415). *The Literal Meaning of Genesis* (*De Genesi ad Literam*). In the Ancient Christian Writers series, No. 41 (1982). Paulist Press. Mahwah, NJ. Pp. 23-27.

Catechisim of the Catholic Church (11 April 2003). Libreria Editrice Vaticana. Nos. 236, 1996, 1999-2000. https://www.vatican.va/archive/ENG0015/_INDEX.HTM

Green, Jay P. (1988). *Pocket Interlinear New Testament*. Baker Book House. Grand Rapids, MI. P. 586.

Hontheim, J. (1910). Heaven. In *The Catholic Encyclopedia*. Robert Appleton Company. New York. http://www.newadvent.org/cathen/07170a.htm

Joyce, George. (1912). The Blessed Trinity. In *The Catholic Encyclopedia*. Robert Appleton Company. http://www.newadvent.org/cathen/15047a.htm

Pohle, Joseph (1910). Justification. In *The Catholic Encyclopedia*. Robert Appleton Company. New York. https://www.newadvent.org/cathen/08573a.htm

Schroeder, H. J. (1978). *The Canons and Decrees of the Council of Trent*. TAN. Rockford, IL. Pp. 31-32.

Sollier, Joseph (1911). Final Perseverance. In *The Catholic Encyclopedia*. Robert Appleton Company. New York. https://www.newadvent.org/cathen/11711a.htm

Chapter 9

About Pregnancy (29 May 2024). Courtesy of the Eunice Kennedy Shriver National Institute of Child Health and Human Development. https://www.nichd.nih.gov/health/topics/pregnancy/conditioninfo

Aquinas, Thomas (1274). *Summa Theologiae*. Supplement to the Third Part, Appendix I. Online edition courtesy of Kevin Knight (2017). https://www.newadvent.org/summa/5.htm

Ben David, Chen, Udi Ergaz, Yaniv Zipori, Ido Solt (February 2025). Ectopic Fallopian Tube Pregnancy Relocation to the Uterine Cavity – Truth or Fiction? Primum non Nocere. *Harefuah*. **164**(2):100-102. Hebrew. https://pubmed.ncbi.nlm.nih.gov/39987478/

Catechisim of the Catholic Church (November 2019). 2nd edition. United States Conference of Catholic Bishops. Nos. 1257, 1261. https://www.usccb.org/sites/default/files/flipbooks/catechism/322/

Cecchino, G.N., Araujo Júnior, E., and Elito Júnior, J. (2014). Methotrexate for Ectopic Pregnancy: When and How. *Arch Gynecol Obstet*. **290**: 417–423. https://doi.org/10.1007/s00404-014-3266-9

CIC (1998). *Code of Canon Law: Latin-English Edition*. Translated by the Canon Law Society of America. P. 286. See also: https://www.vatican.va/archive/cod-iuris-canonici/eng/documents/cic_lib4-cann834-878_en.html

Cleveland Clinic (11 February 2020). *New Ohio Bill Falsely Suggests That Reimplantation of Ectopic Pregnancy Is Possible*. https://consultqd.clevelandclinic.org/new-ohio-bill-falsely-suggests-that-reimplantation-of-ectopic-pregnancy-is-possible

Cleveland Clinic (8 March 2022a). *Uterus*. https://my.clevelandclinic.org/health/body/22467-uterus

Cleveland Clinic (14 November 2022b). *Pregnancy Complications.* https://my.clevelandclinic.org/health/articles/24442-pregnancy-complications

Cleveland Clinic (18 January 2023). *Ectopic Pregnancy.* https://my.clevelandclinic.org/health/diseases/9687-ectopic-pregnancy

Fox, James (1910). Natural Law. In *The Catholic Encyclopedia.* Robert Appleton Company. New York. https://www.newadvent.org/cathen/09076a.htm

Francis, Christina (25 March 2024). The Medical Basis of the Mifepristone Ruling. *The Wall Street Journal.* https://www.wsj.com/articles/the-medical-basis-of-the-mifepristone-ruling-supreme-court-abortion-health-risks-7ef3df6b

Gacek (2009). Conceiving Pregnancy: U.S. Medical Dictionaries and Their Definitions of Conception and Pregnancy. *National Catholic Bioethics Quarterly.* **9**(3): 543-553. https://downloads.frc.org/EF/EF09D12.pdf

Healy, Edwin F. (2025). *Indirect Abortion.* EWTN. https://www.ewtn.com/catholicism/library/indirect-abortion-12081

Hope of Salvation for Infants Who Die Without Being Baptised. https://www.vatican.va/roman_curia/congregations/cfaith/cti_documents/rc_con_cfaith_doc_20070419_un-baptised-infants_en.html#_ftn109

John Hopkins Medicine (2025). *Pregnancy Complications.* https://www.hopkinsmedicine.org/health/conditions-and-diseases/staying-healthy-during-pregnancy/complications-of-pregnancy

Kirk, E., C. Bromley, and T. Bourne (March/April 2014). Diagnosing Ectopic Pregnancy and Current Concepts in the Management of Pregnancy of Unknown Location. *Human Reproduction Update.* **20**(2): 250–261. https://doi.org/10.1093/humupd/dmt047

Lanfranchi, Angela (20 June 2024). *What Catholic Social Teaching Says About the Status of Embryos Part One* https://www.cathmed.org/the-pulse/what-catholic-social-teaching-says-about-the-status-of-embryos/

Miranda, Fred de, and June, Patricia Lee (March 2017). *When Human Life Begins.* Position statement of the American College of Pediatricians. https://acpeds.org/position-statements/when-human-life-begins/

Müller, Gerhard (23 July 2025). Cardinal Müller: German Bishops are Failing to Defend the Unborn due to Political Cowardice. *LifeSiteNews.com.* https://www.lifesitenews.com/analysis/cardinal-muller-german-bishops-are-failing-to-defend-the-unborn-due-to-political-cowardice/

Office on Women's Health (27 February 2025), U.S. Department of Health and Human Services, womenshealth.gov (or girlshealth.gov). *Pregnancy Complications.* https://womenshealth.gov/pregnancy/youre-pregnant-now-what/pregnancy-complications

Ott, Ludwig (May 1960). *Fundamentals of Catholic Dogma.* 4th edition. TAN Books, Rockford, Illinois. Pp. 94-96.

Papageorgiou, Dimitrios, Ioakeim Sapantzoglou, Ioannis Prokopakis, Eleftherios Zachariou (13 June 2025). Tubal Ectopic Pregnancy: From Diagnosis to Treatment. *Biomedicines.* **13**(6): 1465. https://www.mdpi.com/2227-9059/13/6/1465

Pope John Paul II (25 March 1995). *Evangelium Vitae.* Nos. 58, 62-63. https://www.vatican.va/content/john-paul-ii/en/encyclicals/documents/hf_jp-ii_enc_25031995_evangelium-vitae.html

Pope Pius IX (8 December 1854). *Ineffabilis Deus.* https://www.papalencyclicals.net/pius09/p9ineff.htm

Pope Pius XII (12 August 1950). *Humani Generis.* No. 37. https://www.vatican.va/content/pius-xii/en/encyclicals/documents/hf_p-xii_enc_12081950_humani-generis.html

Raine-Bennett, Tina, Fassett, Michael J., et al. (1 August 2022). Disparities in the Incidence of Ectopic Pregnancy in a Large Health Care System in California, 2010–2019. *The Permanente Journal.* **26**(3). https://www.thepermanentejournal.org/doi/10.7812/TPP/21.099

Redinger, Ashley, and Hao Nguyen (12 February 2024). *Incomplete Miscarriage.* National Library of Medicine. Courtesy of StatPearls Publishing. https://www.ncbi.nlm.nih.gov/sites/books/NBK559071/

Rosshirt, Alana M. (May, 1959). How to Baptize in Case of Miscarriage. *Magazine of Catholic Family Living.* https://www.padreperegrino.org/wp-content/uploads/2023/01/Baptize-in-Case-of-Miscarriage.pdf

Sacred Congregation for the Doctrine of the Faith. (18 November 1974). *Declaration on Procured Abortion*. Nos. 12-13, Endnote 19. https://www.vatican.va/roman_curia/congregations/cfaith/documents/rc_con_cfaith_doc_19741118_declaration-abortion_en.html

Sacred Congregation for the Doctrine of the Faith (8 September 2008). *Dignitas Personae*. Nos. 5, 18, 21-23. https://www.vatican.va/roman_curia/congregations/cfaith/documents/rc_con_cfaith_doc_20081208_dignitas-personae_en.html

Sacred Congregation for the Doctrine of the Faith (22 February 1987). *Donum Vitae*. I.1, I.5, II.A.3. https://www.vatican.va/roman_curia/congregations/cfaith/documents/rc_con_cfaith_doc_19870222_respect-for-human-life_en.html

Seeman, Matthew (29 January 2025). Nevada's Cortez Masto Voting No on RFK Jr. After Pressing Him on Emergency Abortion Care. *News3Lv.com*. https://news3lv.com/news/local/nevada-us-sen-catherine-cortez-masto-robert-f-kennedy-jr-hhs-senate-confirmation-hearing-access-to-emergency-abortions-drug-prices

Sharpe, Alfred (1909). Doubt. In *The Catholic Encyclopedia*. Robert Appleton Company. New York. https://www.newadvent.org/cathen/05141a.htm

Shaw, Russell. "Understanding Detachment." 31 July 2016. *The Catholic Thing*.

https://www.thecatholicthing.org/2016/07/31/understanding-detachment/

Sivalingam Vanitha N., W. Colin Duncan, Emma Kirk, et al. (2011). Diagnosis and Management of Ectopic Pregnancy. *Journal of Family Planning and Reproductive Health Care.* **37**: 231-240. https://srh.bmj.com/content/37/4/231

Stickler, Tracy (5 October 2016). *Pregnancy Complications.* Healthline.com. https://www.healthline.com/health/pregnancy/complications-treatments

Thomas, Columba, G. Kevin Donovan, Miguel A. Fernandez, Cara Buskmiller (August, 2023). Efforts to Transfer Ectopic Embryos to the Uterine Cavity: A Systematic Review. *Journal of Obstetrics and Gynaecology Research.* **49**(8): 1991-1999. https://obgyn.onlinelibrary.wiley.com/doi/10.1111/jog.15678

Toner, Patrick (1910). Limbo. In *The Catholic Encyclopedia.* Robert Appleton Company. New York. https://www.newadvent.org/cathen/09256a.htm

University of Rochester Medical Center (2025). *Complications of Pregnancy.* https://www.urmc.rochester.edu/ob-gyn/maternal-fetal-medicine/maternal-care/pregnancy-complications

Vadakekut, Elsa S., David M. Gnugnoli (27 March 2025). Ectopic Pregnancy. In *StatPearls* [Internet]. Treasure Island (FL): StatPearls Publishing. https://www.ncbi.nlm.nih.gov/books/NBK539860/

Wallace, C. J. (1995). Transplantations of Ectopic Pregnancy from Fallopian Tube to Cavity of Uterus. *The Linacre Quarterly.* **62**(1): 9. https://epublications.marquette.edu/lnq/vol62/iss1/9

Chapter 10

Cleveland Clinic (26 December 2022). *Molar Pregnancy.* https://my.clevelandclinic.org/health/diseases/17889-molar-pregnancy

Healy, Edwin F. (1 January 1963). *Medical Ethics.* Loyola University Press. 440 pp.

Healy, Edwin F. (2025). *Indirect Abortion.* EWTN. https://www.ewtn.com/catholicism/library/indirect-abortion-12081

Sacred Congregation for the Doctrine of the Faith. (21 December 2020). *Note on the Morality of Using Some Anti-Covid-19 Vaccines.* https://www.vatican.va/roman_curia/congregations/cfaith/documents/rc_con_cfaith_doc_20201221_nota-vaccini-anticovid_en.html

Texas Amended Statute (19 August 2025). *Life of the Mother Act.* https://capitol.texas.gov/tlodocs/89R/billtext/html/SB00031F.HTM

Texas Statute (1 September 1989). *Texas Abortion Facility Reporting and Licensing Act.* https://statutes.capitol.texas.gov/Docs/HS/htm/HS.245.htm#245.002

Update: COVID-19 Vaccine Candidates and Abortion-Derived Cell Lines (2 June 2021). Courtesy of the Charlotte Lozier Institute. https://lozierinstitute.org/wp-content/uploads/2023/01/CHART-Analysis-of-COVID-19-Vaccines-02June21.pdf

Walsh, Rachel, Anand Sharma (7 February 2022). Extended Survival of a Premature Infant with a Postnatal Diagnosis of Complete Triploidy. *BMJ Case Report*. **15**(2). https://casereports.bmj.com/content/15/2/e244551

YouTube news item (10 July 2025). Posted by "Now This Impact". http://youtube.com/post/UgkxUoZwURdqordeWeHqRkGwNm0gcRwKelcP?si=b6syN-7HdxCiC8v1

Reference Cited in the Appendix

Sullivan, James (1907). The Athanasian Creed. In *The Catholic Encyclopedia*. Robert Appleton Company. New York. https://www.newadvent.org/cathen/02033b.htm

GLOSSARY

Note that some of these terms represent my understanding of their meaning, while others are formally cited for clarity or specificity. References to Wikipedia and Wiktionary are valid at the time of writing. I mention this because these definitions are more representative of popular consensus opinions than of standards useful for all time. In the rare instance that select definitions have changed from when writing first began (early 2023) until it ended, the date of access is included in parentheses. The religious definitions represent my working usage of them for several decades.

Abortion: see "Embryo reduction", "Induced abortion", " Miscarriage ", "Selective abortion", and "Sin of abortion"

Accident (philosophical): "any contingent (i.e., nonessential) relation between an attribute and its subject, a real objective form, or status of things, ...denoting a being whose essential nature it is to inhere in another as in a subject. Accident thus implies inexistence in substance i.e., not as the contained in the container, not as part in the whole, not as a being in time or place, not as effect in cause, not as the known in the knower; but as an inherent entity or mode in a subject." "The accidents cannot be separated thus from the substance; they have their being only in the substance; they are not the substance, but are by their very nature modifications of the substance." (Munnynk, 1912; Siegfried, 1907)

Actual graces: gifts received through God's intervention that assist in the work of sanctification (Catechism of the Catholic Church, nn. 1999-2000)

Adoption: acceptance to raise a child of other parents as the new parents of the child

Adornment: as used in this treatise, adornment is equivalent to content

Advection: the transport in any direction of a property of the atmosphere or hydrosphere

Apostles: twelve men who were taught and sent out by Christ to preach the Gospel to all nations and to heal the afflicted

Apostolic Tradition: all that Jesus Christ said and did that was handed on in non-written form by His Apostles to their successors and from their successors down to us

Artificial insemination: see "*In vivo* fertilization"

Assume (theological): to take on a form, to adopt

Athanasian Creed: symbol of faith possibly from the 6th century that emphasizes the mysteries of the Trinity and the Incarnation

Atheism: denial of the existence or even possibility of God

Atheistic materialist: a person who rejects belief in God, is a moral relativist, and does not believe in the Christian conception of an afterlife

Baptism (sacramental): the sacrament that works with God for the first infusion of sanctifying grace and the theological virtues of faith, hope, and charity into a person not in a state of justification before God; allows membership in the Church

Baptism of blood: attainment of justification through martyrdom for the kingdom of God through faith in Christ

Baptism of desire: attainment of justification by an act of perfect contrition and pure love of God which contains a desire of baptism (Fanning, 1907)

Beatitude: to know God in His essence, i.e., face to face

Bible: a library of sacred books defined by the Catholic Church, inspired by God, and consisting of the Old and New Testaments

Biblical: pertaining to the Bible

Big Bang: a scientific theory about the beginning of the universe

Body (human): the corporeal substance of a human person

Buoyancy: the principle that unless impeded, lower-density materials will rise against gravity through higher-density materials, such as air bubbles rising through water, or will float above the higher density materials, like wood floating in water; also, the force caused by pressure differences that produce this effect

Catechist: a teacher of religious truth and practice

Catholic Public Domain Version: A Catholic Bible translation from the Clementine Vulgate by Ronald L. Conte, published on 28 March 2009, with reference to the Challoner Rheims-Douay version (Conte, 2009)

Catholicism: the religion started by Jesus Christ

Church (the): the brotherhood and society established by Christ to continue His mission of salvation from sin on earth (Joyce, 1908)

Commandments of Moses (613): a compilation by rabbis (Steinsaltz, 2017) of laws found in the Pentateuch (see "613 Commandments" in Wikipedia)

Communicant: the person who receives the Eucharist, usually during Mass

Complication of pregnancy (before childbirth): any medical condition that puts at risk the health or life of a pregnant woman or the unborn child within her

Conception (human): the beginning of a human life; occurs when an egg cell and sperm cell join to create a zygote

Concupiscence: failure to control the passions and the inclination toward inordinate desires, contrary to reason

Conjugal embrace: sexual intercourse within a valid marriage

Conscience: " Conscience is a judgment of reason whereby the human person recognizes the moral quality of a concrete act that he is going to perform, is in the process of performing, or has already completed. ...Moral conscience...enjoins [a man] at the appropriate moment to do good and to avoid evil. It also judges particular choices, approving those that are good and denouncing those that are evil." (Catechism of the Catholic Church, nn. 1777-1778)

Contraception: preclusion of a pregnancy that would result from sexual activity

Convection: the transport in the vertical direction of a property of the atmosphere or hydrosphere

Decalogue: the Ten Commandments, as listed in the Old Testament

Declaration of Independence: a founding document of the United States that includes in its preamble three fundamental rights of man (life, liberty, pursuit of happiness) that exceed the government's ability to set aside or deny because they do not proceed from human government, but from God

De fide: "of the faith"

Delamination (geological): a process whereby part of the lithosphere beneath the earth's crust "peels off" from the remainder above

Deposit of faith: consists of the Apostolic Tradition and Sacred Scripture, as preserved and handed on by the Magisterium of the Church

Deterministic: an effect that results from a cause

Didache: 1st century A.D. teaching of the twelve Apostles of Jesus Christ (Kirby, 2023)

Distinction: as used in this treatise, distinction is equivalent to structure

Divine law: that which is enacted by God and made known to man through revelation (Slater, 1910a)

Divine revelation: "the communication of some truth by God to a rational creature through means which are beyond the ordinary course of nature" (Joyce, 1912)

Dizygotic twins: siblings conceived as two separately fertilized eggs implanted in the uterine wall at the same time

DNA: deoxyribonucleic acid, a large molecule (macromolecule) that carries genetic information for the development and functioning of an organism (Bates, 2025)

Dogma: knowledge revealed by God that occupies the greatest degree of theological certitude in the hierarchy of Catholic truths

Douay Old Testament: Douay translation of the Old Testament of the Bible, Bishop Challoner revision.

Double effect: a principle (Hardon, 1980) by which it is morally permissible to perform a moral act that has two or more outcomes, one good and the other(s) bad (see Chapter 1)

Economic Trinity: the relationship of the Godhead to man, also "all the works by which God reveals himself and communicates his life" (Catechism of the Catholic Church, n. 236)

Ectopic: out of place

Ectopic pregnancy: a type of pregnancy where an embryo is implanted outside the uterus

Egg cell: the female reproductive cell

Elements of true religion: the written word of God; the life of grace; faith, hope, and charity, with the other interior gifts of the Holy Spirit, as well as visible elements (Catechism of the Catholic Church, n. 819); a moral code based on precepts revealed by God

Embryo (human): the first 8 weeks of human life, beginning with the zygote (Lanfranchi, 2024a)

Embryo loss (death): pregnancy loss during the second through eighth week after fertilization (National Library of Medicine, November 1999)

Embryo reduction: "a procedure in which embryos or fetuses in the womb are directly exterminated", "an intentional selective abortion" (Sacred Congregation for the Doctrine of the Faith, 2008)

Embryo transfer: the placement of an embryo into the internal genital tract (specifically the uterine cavity) of a female (Sacred Congregation for the Doctrine of the Faith, 1987)

Embryonic development: the part of the life cycle that begins just after fertilization of the female egg cell by the male sperm cell

Endurance: patient perseverance of the good

ERV: English Revised Version translation of the Bible

Essence: that which a thing is (Aveling, 1909)

Eternal law: the wisdom of God as it governs His creation (Aquinas, 1274a)

Eternity: beyond or outside of time

Ethics: a code of conduct that distinguishes what one ought to do from what one ought not do

Eucharist: Body, Blood, Soul, and Divinity of the Second Person of the Trinity, Jesus Christ, under the species (forms) of bread and wine

Evolution (biological): the change in physical or behavioral characteristics of biological populations that are passed on from parents to offspring over successive generations (National Academy of Sciences, 2025)

Extended family: parents, children, grandparents, aunts, uncles, cousins, etc.

Faith: trust based on experience or reason, a set of beliefs, or more technically a living faith is "an act of the intellect assenting to the truth at the command of the will" (Aquinas, 1274b)

Family: consisting of the nuclear and extended family

Family values (Christian): values taught by Christ and reinforced within a family, which include high moral standards, spiritual responsibilities, and Christian discipline

Family values (secular): "values held to be traditionally taught or reinforced within a family, such as those of high moral standards and discipline" (third definition in Wikipedia, originating in the Oxford Dictionaries)

Fetal death (demise): death of a fetus in the uterus (National Library of Medicine, January 1999)

Fertilization (human): the union of a human egg cell and a human sperm cell

Fertilization age: a measure of the age of a pregnancy taken from the date of fertilization

Fetus: human life beginning in the ninth week after conception (Marcin, 2023, Lanfranchi, 2024a)

Foster care: care of a child by a family member, other legally-responsible person, or institution when the child's parents are unable to supply proper care

Gamete: a reproductive cell

Gene: a unit of hereditary information that determines a specific trait in an organism (Green, 2025a)

General judgment: the judgment of all human persons after Christ returns at the end of the present age

General resurrection: the resurrection from the dead of people's bodies to be rejoined to their souls at the general judgment

Generate: to beget

Genetic: hereditary

Genome: entire set of DNA instructions (all genetic information) of an organism (Green, 2025b)

Gestational age: a measure of the age of a pregnancy taken from the beginning of the woman's last menstrual period

Gestational trophoblastic disease (GTD): a group of pregnancy-related disorders that develop inside the uterus; uterine tumors (Seckl, 2010)

Gift: something freely given without expectation of payment or reciprocity

God: infinite creator of the universe, transcending the universe, eternal, with many limitless attributes such as all powerful, all knowing, unchangeable, perfect justice, boundless mercy, etc.

God the Father: First Person of the Trinity

Godhead: the Trinity of divine persons known as the one God

Good: a free action or conduct that conforms to right reason, or the possession of perfections proper to our nature (Fox, 1909)

Gospel: a written record of Christ's words and deeds, with commentary by the Gospel authors

Grace: a free and undeserved assistance from God (noun), or to supply this assistance (verb)

Heritable: traits that are able to be passed on from parents to offspring

Holy Ghost: older name of the Holy Spirit

Holy Spirit: Third Person of the Trinity

Human being/human life: an individual substance of a human nature, consisting of a physical body and a spiritual soul

Human nature: to act as a human being acts; among these active abilities are: to reason, to choose prudential and moral courses of action, to generate new human beings, to live in community, to seek after and serve God

Human person: a human being of body and soul created by God

Human zygote: a successfully fertilized human egg which initiates embryonic development (Johnson, 1995)

Hydatidiform mole (complete): a tumor in which a nonviable fertilized egg without female genetic material implants in the uterus; a type of gestational trophoblastic disease that is not a pregnancy because there is no embryo (Jacobson, 2024; Cavaliere, 2009; The Miscarriage Association, 2025)

Hydatidiform mole (partial): nonviable fertilization with double the male genetic material that in very rare instances can result in an abnormal pregnancy (Jacobson, 2024; Cavaliere, 2009; The Miscarriage Association, 2025)

Hypostatic union: "a theological term used with reference to the Incarnation to express the revealed truth that in Christ one person subsists in two natures, the divine and the human" (Pace, 1910)

Immaculate Conception (Catholic dogma): Mary, the mother of Jesus, was preserved from the privation of sanctifying grace (i.e., original sin) from the moment of her conception in her mother's womb

Implantation (normal uterine): attachment of an early-stage embryo to the wall of the uterus

Incarnation of God: the act by which the Second Person of the Trinity assumed (took on) the body of a man, and the ongoing reality of this union between the eternal Divine and the human

Induced abortion (direct, procured): the direct termination of a pregnancy, from conception to birth, with the intent to destroy a human life, "every act tending directly to destroy human life in the womb". In the context of pregnancy, "procured abortion is the deliberate and direct killing, by whatever means it is carried out, of a human being in the initial phase of his or her existence, extending from conception to birth". ..."I declare that direct abortion, that is, abortion willed as an end or as a means, always constitutes a grave moral disorder, since it is the deliberate killing of an innocent human being" (Pope John Paul II, 1995).

Infused knowledge: natural and divine knowledge gifted to Adam and Eve by God

Intention: a commitment of the will to a particular course of action or belief

In vitro: outside a living organism in an artificial environment

In vitro extermination: the destruction of human embryos outside of a woman's body in an artificial environment

In vitro fertilization: an artificial fertilization of a female egg by instrumental intervention outside of the female's body

In vivo fertilization: an artificial fertilization of a female egg by instrumental intervention inside of the female's body

Isostasy: buoyant equilibrium between the lithosphere and the deformable upper mantle below

Justice (virtue of): a moral quality or habit which perfects the will and inclines it to render to each and to all what belongs to them (Slater, 1910b)

Justification: the remission of sins and "the sanctification and renewal of the inward man through the voluntary reception of" grace and other gifts such as the supernatural virtues of faith, hope, and charity (Schroeder, 1978)

Kingdom of God: the reign of God's justice everywhere that people allow themselves to be ruled by Christ's will for mankind

Legal person: a person recognized as having civil rights before the civil law

Life: an animate, vital good created by God to serve Him in its own way

Lifeform: a category of an animate, vital organism

Lithosphere: the outer sphere of the earth that consists of the combination of the earth's crust and rigid upper mantle

Logos: Second Person of the Trinity, also known as the Son, or Word, of God

Macroevolution: a popular consensus paradigm in biology that life becomes increasingly complex over time through processes found in nature

Magisterium: the organ in the Church "of preservation and transmission of traditional and revealed truth" (Bainvel, 1912), less formally considered the teaching authority of the Church

Material: temporal, not spiritual

Matter (normal or ordinary): matter that is made up of atoms and their constituent particles

Medical condition: disordered health status such as illness, disease, disability, injury

Medical oath: basic principles for medical professionals that include a code of conduct

Merit: something worthy or deserving of reward

Microevolution: small-scale changes within species that are easily observable, such as changes in traits

Miracle: supernatural manifestation of God's will

Miscarriage: the spontaneous natural termination of a pregnancy resulting in the loss of an embryo or fetus from the uterus during the first 20 weeks of gestational age, sometimes strangely called a "spontaneous abortion" (Medical News Today, 2018; MedlinePlus, 2025)

Molar pregnancy: see "Hydatidiform mole"; a complete hydatidiform mole is not a pregnancy

Monozygotic twins: siblings conceived from a single fertilized egg that divides into two separate embryos; occurs from 0-14 days after fertilization (Hall, 2003; Jonsson, 2021)

Morality: recognition of the distinction between good and evil or between right and wrong according to God's standard

Motive: an incentive or reason to act in a particular way

Murder: the unjust taking of an innocent human life

Mutagenesis: generation of a mutation

Mutation: any change in the sequence of an organism's genetic information or the process by which the changes occur (Fitzgerald, 2019)

Mystery (sacred): public religious knowledge not fully apprehensible nor explainable by science or philosophy

NAB: New American Bible translation of the Bible

Narrative: a real or fictional story proffered by a narrator

Natural: of or pertaining to the physical universe

Natural Family Planning: a method of spacing births by using the natural fertility cycle of a woman

Natural law: "the rational creature's participation [in] the eternal law" (Aquinas, 1274c); the rule of conduct prescribed to us by our Creator in the nature He has endowed us and "manifested to us by the purely natural medium of reason" (Fox, 1910). "The natural moral law expresses and lays down the purposes, rights and duties which are based upon the bodily and spiritual nature of the human person. ...defined as the rational order whereby man is called by the Creator to direct and regulate his life and actions and in particular to make use of his own body" (Sacred Congregation for the Doctrine of the Faith, 1987).

Nature (environment): the physical world

Nature (practical): the cause of a thing's behavior

New Testament: a library of sacred books defined by the Catholic Church, inspired by God, and written after the death of Jesus Christ

Nicene Creed: a statement of Catholic belief first adopted at the ecumenical Council of Nicaea in 325 and finalized in 381 at the ecumenical Council of Constantinople (Wilhelm, 1911)

Nonviable: the inability of a fetus to survive outside of the womb (cf. Pettker, 2023)

NRSV: New Revised Standard translation of the Bible

Nuclear family: a mother and father validly married in the eyes of God, and their children

Offspring: a person's children or descendants

Old Testament: a library of sacred books defined by the Catholic Church, inspired by God, and written prior to the birth of Jesus Christ

Ontological Trinity: the relationship of the persons of the Trinity to one another

Original sin: the sin of disobedience committed by Adam, as prompted by Eve, in the Garden of Eden, the effects thereof being transmitted by human procreation

Particular judgment: the judgment by God that each man undergoes at the moment of physical death

Person: "an individual substance of a rational nature" (Boethius, 520), applies only to created beings with intellect and will

Persons of the Trinity (divine): "The three Divine realities are relations, each identified with the Divine Essence" (Geddes, 1911), or the Godhead: God the Father, God the Son, God the Holy Spirit.

Phenotype: all of an organism's traits (National Human Genome Research Institute, 2025)

Photon: a tiny packet of energy, such as light

Pregnancy: the condition of carrying developing offspring within a woman's body (cf. Lanfranchi, 2024a; Lanfranchi 2024b)

Procreation (human): the process by which a human person produces others of its biological kind; also known as co-creation with God of a human person

Pro-life: commitment to the protection of all human life, from conception to proper upbringing, education, adult life, and natural death

Proximate: close or adjacent

Public revelation: Biblical scripture and the Apostolic Tradition, the fullness of which is a divine person, Jesus Christ

Radiation: the emission or transmission of energy, such as light, through space or materials

Randomness: apparent or actual lack of purpose, predictability, or order in information or sequence (cf. Wiktionary and Wikipedia)

Refulgence: divine light, an aspect of divine presence perceived as light

Remote: distant

Reproduction (sexual): the biological process by which offspring are generated from their parents

Rheims New Testament: Rheims translation of the New Testament of the Bible, Bishop Challoner revision.

Rheology: the discipline that studies the deformation and flow of solids and liquids

Righteous: just in the eyes of God

Righteousness: to be righteous

Sacred Scripture: the Bible, a collection of books determined by Christ's Church to contain the inspired writings of divine revelation as known through the history of men

Saint: a person who lives a sinless life on earth or who lives in heaven

Salvation: a present hope in full adoption as children of God to live in a future heavenly world where redeemed souls join back with their own bodies, which are transformed to be capable of living in the heavenly world

Sanctification: the perfection of a man's soul that enables him to live with God and to act righteously (Catechism of the Catholic Church, nn. 1999-2000)

Sanctifying (habitual) grace: a participation in the life of God, a mysterious sharing in the internal life of God (the Ontological Trinity)

Scholar: a learned person and proven thinker

Selective abortion: applying specifically to embryos, "the deliberate and direct elimination of one or more innocent human beings in the initial phase of their existence" (Sacred Congregation for the Doctrine of the Faith, 2008)

Selective breeding: breeding within a species to produce an engineered outcome, a sort of human-induced microevolution that changes traits within a species

Sex: male or female

Sin of abortion: "the deliberate and direct killing, by whatever means it is carried out, of a human being in the initial phase of his or her existence, extending from conception to birth" (Sacred Congregation for the Doctrine of the Faith, 2008), includes the destruction of embryos outside of a woman's body in an artificial environment.

Solar wind: streams of charged particles constantly emitted by the sun

Son of God: refers to God the Son, the Second Person of the Trinity, when "Son" is capitalized

Soul (human): the spiritual substance of a human person

Species (biological): for purposes of this treatise, living things that can produce fertile offspring when mating

Sperm: the male reproductive cell

Spirit: a living substance that is not material

Stillbirth: the spontaneous natural termination of a pregnancy resulting in the loss of an embryo or fetus from the uterus after 20 weeks of gestational age and before birth (U.S. Centers for Disease Control and Prevention, 2025)

Subject: an observer, or a being capable of subjective experiences, consciousness, or relationship (cf. Wiktionary and Wikipedia)

Substance (philosophical): "Nothing is more evident than that things change. It is impossible for anything to be twice in absolutely the same state; on the other hand all the changes are not equally profound. Some appear to be purely external: a piece of wood may be hot or cold, lying flat or upright, yet it is still wood; but if it be completely burnt so as to be transformed into ashes and gases, it is no longer wood; the specific, radical characteristics by which we describe wood have totally disappeared. Thus there are two kinds of changes: one affects the radical characteristics of things, and consequently determines the existence or non-existence of these things; the other in no way destroys these characteristics, and so, while modifying the thing, does not affect it fundamentally. It is necessary, therefore, to recognize in each thing certain secondary realities (see *accident*) and also a permanent *fundamentum* which continues to exist notwithstanding the superficial changes, which serves as a basis or support for the secondary realities — what, in a word, we term the substance. Its fundamental characteristic is to be in itself and by itself, and not in another subject as accidents are." (Munnynk, 1912)

Supernatural: transcending nature

Tanakh: the Hebrew Bible

Telos (τέλος): aim or goal

Temporal: in time, in the world

Temporal sphere: of or relating to time and the material world, as opposed to the sacred or the eternal (cf. Wiktionary)

Traditional values: beliefs, morals, and principles passed down through generations

Trait: an observable characteristic of an organism, such as blue or brown eyes (Hull, 2025)

Trinity: the three persons in the divine Godhead (God the Father, God the Son, God the Holy Spirit)

True religion (beginning with Christ): the religion established by Jesus Christ, but existing in nascent or less integral beliefs ever since Adam and Eve were first created to know, love, and serve God

True religion (pre-Christian): the religion revealed by God to Adam and Eve, handed down to the early patriarchs, and eventually revealed again to Moses and the prophets of the Old Testament

Twins: two offspring produced by the same pregnancy

Tubal pregnancy: *an attempt at pregnancy* where an early-stage embryo implants inside a Fallopian tube; a misnomer because it is not a true pregnancy

Unintended pregnancy loss: miscarriage, embryo death (loss), fetal demise, hydatidiform mole, ectopic pregnancy, others (AAPC, 2025)

U.S. Constitution: a founding document of the United States that limits the imposition of government on people's lives

Uterus: an organ of the female reproductive system in which the young are conceived and develop until birth

Vainglory: excessive vanity; included under the deadly sin of pride

Viable (pregnancy): a fetus or embryo with a detectable heartbeat (Pettker, 2023), or an embryo that can develop to survive outside of the womb

Viability (fetal): the ability of a fetus to survive outside of the womb (Pettker, 2023)

Vice: a habit inclining one to sin (Delany, 1912)

Virtue: a good habit consonant with our nature (Waldron, 1912)

Woman: a human person born with the procreative capability of a human female

Womb: uterus

World: temporal existence

Zygote: a fertilized egg cell, formed when an egg cell and sperm cell join to create a new unique organism

REFERENCES CITED IN THE GLOSSARY

AAPC (2025). *Pregnancy with Abortive Outcome.* https://www.aapc.com/codes/icd-10-codes-range/O00-O9A/O00-O08/

Aquinas, Thomas (1274a). *Summa Theologiae* I-II.93.1. Online edition courtesy of Kevin Knight (2017). https://www.newadvent.org/summa/2093.htm

Aquinas, Thomas (1274b). *Summa Theologiae* II-II.4.5. Online edition courtesy of Kevin Knight (2017). https://www.newadvent.org/summa/3004.htm

Aquinas, Thomas (1274c). *Summa Theologiae* I-II.91.2. Online edition courtesy of Kevin Knight (2017). https://www.newadvent.org/summa/2091.htm

Aveling, Francis (1909). Essence and Existence. In *The Catholic Encyclopedia*. Robert Appleton Company. New York. https://www.newadvent.org/cathen/05543b.htm

Bainvel, Joseph (1912). Tradition and Living Magisterium. In *The Catholic Encyclopedia*. Robert Appleton Company. New York. http://www.newadvent.org/cathen/15006b.htm

Bates, Sarah A. (11 May 2025). *Deoxyribonucleic Acid (DNA)*. Public domain. National Human Genome Research Institute. https://www.genome.gov/genetics-glossary/Deoxyribonucleic-Acid-DNA

Boethius (circa 520). *Liber De Persona et Duabus Naturis Contra Eutychen Et Nestorium*. Chapter III. Courtesy of biblehub.com. https://biblehub.com/library/boethius/the_theological_tractates/a_treatise_against_eutyches_and.htm#1

Catechisim of the Catholic Church (11 April 2003). Libreria Editrice Vaticana. Nos. 236, 819, 1777-1778, 1999-2000. https://www.vatican.va/archive/ENG0015/_INDEX.HTM

Cavaliere, Alessandro, Santina Ermito, Angela Dinatale, Rosa Pedata (January-March 2009). Management of Molar Pregnancy. *Journal of Prenatal Medicine*. **3**(1): 15-17 https://pmc.ncbi.nlm.nih.gov/articles/PMC3279094/

Conte, Ronald L. (28 March 2009). *The Catholic Public Domain Version of the Sacred Bible*. https://www.sacredbible.org/catholic/version.htm

Delany, Joseph (1912). Vice. In *The Catholic Encyclopedia*. Robert Appleton Company. New York. http://www.newadvent.org/cathen/08571c.htm

Fanning, William (1907). Baptism. In *The Catholic Encyclopedia*. Robert Appleton Company. New York. https://www.newadvent.org/cathen/02258b.htm

Fitzgerald, Devon M., and Susan M. Rosenberg (1 April 2019). What is Mutation? A chapter in the series: How Microbes "Jeopardize" the Modern Synthesis. *PLOS Genetics*. **15**(4). https://doi.org/10.1371/journal.pgen.1007995

Fox, James (1909). Good. In *The Catholic Encyclopedia*. Robert Appleton Company. New York. https://www.newadvent.org/cathen/06636b.htm

Fox, James (1910). Natural Law. In *The Catholic Encyclopedia*. Robert Appleton Company. New York. https://www.newadvent.org/cathen/09076a.htm

Geddes, Leonard (1911). Person. In *The Catholic Encyclopedia*. Robert Appleton Company. New York. http://www.newadvent.org/cathen/11726a.htm

Green, Eric (14 May 2025a). *Gene*. National Human Genome Research Institute. https://www.genome.gov/genetics-glossary/Genome

Green, Eric (14 May 2025b). *Genome*. National Human Genome Research Institute. https://www.genome.gov/genetics-glossary/Genome

Hall, Judith G. (30 August 2003). Twinning. *The Lancet*. **362**(9385): 735-743. https://doi.org/10.1016/S0140-6736(03)14237-7

Hardon, John A. (1980). *Modern Catholic Dictionary*. Doubleday. Garden City, NY. P. 171.

Hull, Sarah Chandros (14 May 2025). *Trait*. National Human Genome Research Institute. https://www.genome.gov/genetics-glossary/Trait

Jacobson, John G. (15 October 2024). *Hydatidiform mole*. Medline Plus. https://medlineplus.gov/ency/article/000909.htm

Johnson, M. (1995). Delayed Hominization: Reflections on Some Recent Catholic Claims for Delayed Hominization. *Theological Studies*. **56**(4): 743–763. https://doi.org/10.1177/004056399505600407. Public domain viewing at: *The Free Library*. Quaestio Disputata: Delayed Hominization, Reflections on Some Recent Catholic Claims for Delayed Hominization. https://www.thefreelibrary.com/Quaestio+Disputata%3a+delay

ed+hominization%2c+reflections+on+some+recent...-a017924051

Jonsson, Hakon, Erna Magnusdottir, Hannes P. Eggertsson, et al. (2021). Differences Between Germline Genomes of Monozygotic Twins. *Nature Genetics.* **53**: 27–34. https://doi.org/10.1038/s41588-020-00755-1

Joyce, George (1908). The Church. In *The Catholic Encyclopedia.* Robert Appleton Company. New York. https://www.newadvent.org/cathen/03744a.htm

Joyce, George (1912). Revelation. In *The Catholic Encyclopedia.* Robert Appleton Company. New York. https://www.newadvent.org/cathen/13001a.htm

Kirby, Peter (2023). The Didache. *Early Christian Writings.* http://www.earlychristianwritings.com/text/didache-roberts.html

Lanfranchi, Angela (20 June 2024a). *What Catholic Social Teaching Says About the Status of Embryos Part One.* https://www.cathmed.org/the-pulse/what-catholic-social-teaching-says-about-the-status-of-embryos/

Lanfranchi, Angela (15 July 2024b). *What Catholic Social Teaching Says About the Status of Embryos Part Two.* https://www.cathmed.org/the-pulse/what-catholic-social-teaching-says-about-the-status-of-embryos/

Marcin, Ashely (12 April 2023). *Embryo vs. Fetus: Fetal Development Week-by-Week.* Healthline.com. https://www.healthline.com/health/pregnancy/embryo-fetus-development

Medical News Today (28 June 2018). *Miscarriage: What You Need to Know.* https://www.medicalnewstoday.com/articles/262941

MedlinePlus (2 July 2025). *Miscarriage.* https://medlineplus.gov/miscarriage.html

Munnynk, Mark Mary de (1912). Substance. In *The Catholic Encyclopedia.* Robert Appleton Company. New York. https://www.newadvent.org/cathen/14322c.htm

National Academy of Sciences (2025). Definition of "evolution", under *Definitions of Evolutionary Terms.* https://www.nationalacademies.org/evolution/definitions

National Human Genome Research Institute (20 July 2025). *Phenotype.* https://www.genome.gov/genetics-glossary/Phenotype

National Library of Medicine (3 November 1999). *Embryo Loss.* https://www.ncbi.nlm.nih.gov/mesh/?term=Embryo+loss

National Library of Medicine (1 January 1999). *Fetal Deth.* https://www.ncbi.nlm.nih.gov/mesh/?term=Embryo+loss

Pace, Edward. (1910). Hypostatic Union. In *The Catholic Encyclopedia.* Robert Appleton Company. New York. http://www.newadvent.org/cathen/07610b.htm

Pettker, Christian M.; Mark A. Turrentine; Hyagriv N. Simhan (4 August 2023). The Limits of Viability. *Obstetrics and Gynecology.* **142**(3): 725-726. https://journals.lww.com/greenjournal/fulltext/2023/09000/the_limits_of_viability.29.aspx

Pope John Paul II (25 March 1995). *Evangelium Vitae.* Nos. 58, 62. https://www.vatican.va/content/john-paul-ii/en/encyclicals/documents/hf_jp-ii_enc_25031995_evangelium-vitae.html

Sacred Congregation for the Doctrine of the Faith (8 September 2008). *Dignitas Personae*. Nos. 21-23. https://www.vatican.va/roman_curia/congregations/cfaith/documents/rc_con_cfaith_doc_20081208_dignitas-personae_en.html

Sacred Congregation for the Doctrine of the Faith (22 February 1987). *Donum Vitae*. I.5, II. https://www.vatican.va/roman_curia/congregations/cfaith/documents/rc_con_cfaith_doc_19870222_respect-for-human-life_en.html

Schroeder, H. J. (1978). *The Canons and Decrees of the Council of Trent*. TAN. Rockford, IL. P. 33.

Seckl, Michael J., Neil J Sebire, Ross S Berkowitz (28 August 2010). Gestational Trophoblastic Disease. *The Lancet*. **376** (9742) 717-729. Published online 29 July 2010 at https://doi.org/10.1016/S0140-6736(10)60280-2

Siegfried, Francis (1907). Accident. In *The Catholic Encyclopedia*. Robert Appleton Company. New York. https://www.newadvent.org/cathen/01096c.htm

Slater, Thomas (1910a). Moral Aspect of Divine Law. In *The Catholic Encyclopedia*. Robert Appleton Company. New York. http://www.newadvent.org/cathen/09071a.htm

Slater, Thomas (1910b). Justice. In *The Catholic Encyclopedia*. Robert Appleton Company. New York. http://www.newadvent.org/cathen/08571c.htm

Steinsaltz, Adin (15 October 2017). *Koren Talmud Bavli: Noe Edition*. Volume 31: Makkot Shevuot (23b and 24a). The William Davidson digital edition.

https://www.sefaria.org/Makkot.23b.18?lang=bi&with=all&lang2=en

The Miscarriage Association (January 2025). *Molar Pregnancy (Hydatidiform Mole).* https://www.miscarriageassociation.org.uk/wp-content/uploads/2017/12/Molar-Pregnancy.pdf

U.S. Centers for Disease Control and Prevention (26 August 2025). *About Stillbirth.* https://www.cdc.gov/stillbirth/about/index.html

Waldron, Martin Augustine (1912). Virtue. In *The Catholic Encyclopedia.* Robert Appleton Company. New York. https://www.newadvent.org/cathen/15472a.htm

Wilhelm, Joseph (1911). Nicene Creed. In *The Catholic Encyclopedia.* Robert Appleton Company. New York. https://www.newadvent.org/cathen/11049a.htm

About the Author

Randal Mandock enjoyed two parallel careers for most of his working life: physical scientist and religious educator. His formal technical education includes geology, geophysics, health physics, and atmospheric sciences, graduating with a Ph.D. from the Georgia Institute of Technology. His training in religion encompasses the first year of formation for the Catholic diaconate, advanced certification in catechesis, and qualification in biblical creationism from the Institute for Creation Research. Dr. Mandock served as an associate professor in the Department of Physics at Clark Atlanta University, a geophysicist for two oil companies, a science teacher, and a scientific researcher and contractor. His career in religion spanned more than four decades as a catechist, internet apologist, and director of religious education at a Catholic parish. He is a member of St. Stephen the Martyr parish in Lilburn, Georgia, and was discharged honorably from the USMC with the rank of sergeant.

Dr. Mandock decided to write this book as an advocacy for a redefinition of terms relating to pregnancy and its complications. He considered this necessary because of the confusion among many about the scope of the challenges to the birth of babies in modern societies. For far too long those who would terminate unborn children have had control of the narrative about pregnancy and its ending. This book is an attempt to revise that narrative to make it more favorable to the preservation of children in their mother's womb.

www.ingramcontent.com/pod-product-compliance
Lightning Source LLC
LaVergne TN
LVHW040220110826
845146LV00005B/1349

9798888704103